ATI TEAS® Study Manual

FOR THE TEST OF ESSENTIAL ACADEMIC SKILLS

Contributors/Reviewers

Angela Broaddus, PhD Curriculum & Instruction

George Christoph, M.Ed. Mathematics, NBCT

Shauna Hedgepeth, MS Science Education

Deidre Meyer, MS Instructional Design

Joe Meyer, BS Mathematics, NBCT

Suzanne Myers, MS Curriculum & Instruction

Derek Prater, MS Journalism

Vidya Rajan, PhD Genetics

Kris Shaw, MS Education

Charlotte Waters, MS Science Education

Director of content development: Derek Prater

Project management: Janet Hines

Copy editing: Kelly Von Lunen, Derek Prater

Layout: Randi Hardy, Spring Lenox

Illustrations: Randi Hardy

Cover design: Jason Buck

Interior book design: Spring Lenox

Table of contents

MATHEMATICS 63

Number and algebra

Measurement and data

SCIENCE 105

Human anatomy and physiology

ENGLISH AND LANGUAGE USAGE   163

Introduction

Welcome to the ATI TEAS® Study Manual, your definitive guide to successful preparation for the Test of Essential Academic Skills (TEAS). This book provides the best insight on what type of content will be included on the TEAS and how to most effectively prepare yourself for the test. This is, however, a study *guide*. It should not be the only resource used in your studies. The TEAS covers a broad range of essential skills in reading, mathematics, science, and English and language usage that you should have developed over the course of your academic career. To brush up on those skills, you might need to consult old class notes, textbooks, and authoritative online sources for additional practice and information. This study guide, though, will provide the map to your success. It will provide you with the critical information you need to know about the test itself, an overview of the various objectives covered in each section of the TEAS, examples of the type of content covered for each objective, and practice opportunities for answering questions about each objective.

The test

First, let's cover the essential information you need to know about the TEAS. This test was developed for health science schools to evaluate the academic preparedness of prospective students. Each question on the TEAS is mapped to one of 65 objectives, all of which address topics presented in grades 7 to 12. The objectives assessed are those that health science educators deemed most appropriate and relevant to measure entry-level skills and abilities of health science program applicants. The objectives cover the academic content areas of:

· Reading

· Mathematics

· Science

· English and language usage

The detailed test plan, which includes examples of knowledge, skills, and abilities for each objective, is covered by the chapters of this manual. Keep in mind that the examples for each objective are not comprehensive of all the content that could be covered for that objective. If you focus on these, you'll likely be in good shape, but any content that fits the described objective is fair game for inclusion on the TEAS.

The TEAS is composed of 170 questions, 20 of which are unscored pretest items. Thus, the number of scored questions on which you will be evaluated is 150. These questions are all four-option, multiple-choice questions, and the test is available in both paper-pencil and computer-administered formats. While questions from the four content areas are grouped separately, the TEAS is a single test that provides a composite score based on a given administration. The table below provides the number of questions and time limits for each section of the TEAS.

Content Area	Number of Questions	Time Limit
Reading	53	64 minutes
Mathematics	36	54 minutes
Science	53	63 minutes
English and language usage	28	28 minutes
Total	**170**	**209 minutes**

The objectives are further organized by sub-content areas within each content area, and there are a specified number of scored items for each topic as follows. The number of pretest items per section is not specified by topic.

Content and sub-content areas	Number of scored items	
Reading	**47**	*plus 6 pretest items*
Key ideas and details	22	
Craft and structure	14	
Integration of knowledge and ideas	11	
Mathematics	**32**	*plus 4 pretest items*
Number and algebra	23	
Measurement and data	9	
Science	**47**	*plus 6 pretest items*
Human anatomy and physiology	32	
Life and physical sciences	8	
Scientific reasoning	7	
English and language usage	**24**	*plus 4 pretest items*
Conventions of standard English	9	
Knowledge of language	9	
Vocabulary acquisition	6	

Test administration

Here's what you need to know about taking the test. The TEAS is administered in a standardized environment overseen by a proctor. The proctor will ensure that all testing protocols are strictly enforced.

What to bring

Photo ID: To be admitted to your testing session, you will need to present proper photo identification, such as a driver's license, passport, or green card. You will not be admitted to test if your ID does not meet the following requirements: government-issued, current photograph, examinee signature, and permanent address. A credit card photo or a student ID does not meet the criteria.

Writing instrument: Two sharpened No. 2 pencils with attached erasers. No other writing instruments are allowed.

ATI log-in information: If you are taking the online version, you will need to create a student account at www.atitesting.com prior to test day and have your login information with you.

What not to bring

Plan ahead and leave the following items at home or in your car, as they are not permitted in the exam room.

Additional apparel, including but not limited to jackets, coats, hats, and sunglasses. Discretionary allowances are made for religious apparel. All apparel is subject to inspection by a proctor.

Personal items of any sort, including but not limited to purses, computer bags, backpacks, and duffel bags.

Electronics of any kind, including but not limited to cell phones, smart phones, beepers/pagers, and digital and smart watches.

Food or drink, unless it is documented as a medically necessary item.

What to expect

Testing staff will check your photo ID, admit you to your test room, and direct you to a seat.

Physically present proctors in the room are monitoring for odd or disruptive behavior. Do not engage in misconduct or disruption. If you do, you will be dismissed and your exam will not be scored.

A four-function calculator will be provided by the testing center. You will not be allowed to use calculators that have built-in functionalities or other special features.

The proctor will provide you with scratch paper for use during the test. Scratch paper is not to be used before the exam or during breaks. All paper, in its entirety, must be returned to the proctor at the end of the testing session.

After the Mathematics section, you may take a 10-minute break. During the break, DO NOT access any personal items.

If you need to leave your seat at any time other than the break, raise your hand. Time for the exam section will not stop. Time lost cannot be made up.

If, during the exam, you have a technical issue with your computer, or for any reason need the proctor, raise your hand.

Test challenges or testing room complaints should be reported to the proctor before leaving the room on exam day.

The study manual

This guide is organized based on the test plan for the TEAS to help you target your studies for success on the test. There's a section for each content area, and a chapter for each objective. Each chapter provides an overview of the objective, including the most important concepts included within the examples of knowledge, skills, and abilities. Chapters also include key terms and definitions, study recommendations, practice questions, and study exercises. A key for the practice questions is provided at the end of each topic, so that you can compare your answers and gather additional information from the rationales provided. At the end of each section, there is a quiz that matches the number of the scored items from the test plan. These quizzes provide an excellent practice opportunity, as they have been developed using essentially the same guidelines as the TEAS itself. A key with detailed rationales follows each quiz.

If you use this study manual to thoroughly familiarize yourself with each of the TEAS objectives, to practice answering TEAS-style questions, and to guide your additional studies on the concepts covered here, you will be well on your way to success on the TEAS.

The online practice TEAS

Two online practice versions of the TEAS are available for purchase. These are developed using the same test plan as the proctored versions and provide both the opportunity for additional practice answering TEAS-style questions and for assessing your readiness to take the TEAS successfully. Each of these tests contains 150 items, all of which are scored. The testing interface is similar to that of the online proctored version, except that rationales are provided for each question to further your learning. Upon completing the online practice test, a score report will appear with your results and a list of topics to review. The list of topics to review corresponds to the objectives in the test plan and study manual and indicates the areas on which you should focus your studies.

TEAS scores

Upon completion of the online version of the test, your test will be scored immediately, allowing you to view your TEAS score report at that time. If you took a paper-pencil version of the TEAS, ATI will score the test within 48 hours of receiving it from the testing site. The score report includes your total and content area scores. In addition, the report identifies specific topic areas you missed along with information on where in the study manual you can review the content.

You can access your ATI TEAS score report at any time through your ATI account under My Results. Within that same area, next to your score report, you have the ability to create a Focused Review. A Focused Review is an online review tool that aligns question topics missed and the relevant study manual pages for your review.

"How do I submit my TEAS score to the health science program I am applying to?" you might wonder. If you tested on-site at the program you are applying to, your TEAS transcript is already available to them. If you want to send your transcript to a different program, visit www.atitesting.com/ati_store/ to purchase and send an official TEAS transcript to the program of your choice.

Feedback

All feedback is welcome: suggestions for improvement, reports of mistakes (small or large), and testimonials of effectiveness. Please address feedback to comments@atitesting.com.

ATI TEAS
preparation strategies

When should you start studying for the test? Evidence suggests that you should begin studying well ahead of time so that you can continuously review the material and store the information in your long-term vs. short-term memory[1]. Planning to review your notes, write mock exams, and develop concept maps are just a few strategic examples of ways to plan effective study time[2]. Research suggests that if you have a plan with study goals, study repeatedly over time, and keep track of your learning (self-regulate), your performance will improve[3]. Studying with peers and constantly asking yourself questions about materials, such as "How could I explain this to someone?" or "How does this apply to my life or other information I have learned?", can also help you learn the material[4].

Use the following worksheet to help you prepare for the test. Adapt the sheet to meet your individual needs.

Preparing for the test

The TEAS test is on the following date and time:	
The most important areas for me to study are:	
My top four goals for studying	*I can find or create practice questions at the following places or with the following people.*
1.	1.
2.	2.
3.	3.
4.	
Resources I will use for studying	*Days and times I have set aside exclusively for studying for this test*
1.	Mondays:
2.	Tuesdays:
3.	Wednesdays:
4.	Thursdays:
Concepts or examples I don't understand and need to ask someone about	Fridays:
1.	Saturdays:
2.	Sundays:
3.	
4.	

1. Kornell, 2009; Kitsantas, 2002; Terry 2006
2. Tinnesz, Ahun, & Kiener, 2006
3. Kistantas, 2002
4. van Blerkom, van Blerkom, & Bertsch, 2006; Roberts, 2008; Weinstein, Ridley, Dahl, & Weber, 1988

Where and when to study

The right place and time to study is different for different people. You might prefer to study in a quiet library, in the comfort of your own home, or perhaps in a bustling coffee shop. While it is important to choose a location in which you are comfortable, you must ask yourself whether the spot you chose is an effective study site. As such, a balance between preference and practicality must be struck when deciding where to study. A similar balance must be found when deciding when to study. Although your schedule might restrict the time of day you can study, you should try to study when you are most alert.

Tips

- **Use decent lighting**. Ensure that your study area has adequate lighting. This will keep you from straining while you read your material, in addition to helping you stay awake and alert.

- **Study in a room with a comfortable temperature.** You do not want your study environment to be too hot or too cold. A cooler room temperature is preferable to one that is excessively warm because warm temperatures can promote sleepiness.

- **Have plenty of space.** Your study area should provide ample space for you to organize your study materials in an orderly manner. Everything you need should be easily accessible without requiring a great deal of maneuvering.

- **Avoid distractions.** Try to study in a place with few external distractions. The more focused you are during your studying, the more productive you will be.

- **Study during your alert times.** If you are a morning person, get up early in the morning and study. If you are an evening person, study at night. In either case, make sure you allow yourself to get a good night's sleep.

- **Rearrange other activities.** If extracurricular activities, such as jobs or athletics, take up a lot of your time, try to rearrange your activities so that you can study at your most alert times. Otherwise, determine which days of the week you can study at your most alert times and do so.

Using reading strategies as you read the study manual

Developing strategies for effectively reading texts is key to being successful. Finding strategies to help you read and process a large amount of information is necessary. Research suggests you should try to apply or connect the new information you are reading about to prior information[5]. When reading the material, research also suggests that you scan the material for key words and make sure you are taking good notes on the material[6]. The more organized your approach for the reading, the more successful you will be at remembering what you have read.

Tips

- **Review the text.** Before delving into the details of a reading, scan through the introduction, summary, key terms and definitions, and any stated learning objectives.

- **Outline the text.** You might choose to outline the text on a separate sheet of paper or write in the text directly. Highlighting these parts of the reading will help get you focused on the content and what to expect from the text.

- **Underline topic sentences.** This will help you remember the important concepts when you review the text. It will also help you keep focused while you're reading.

- **Write vocabulary words, concepts, and dates in the margin.** Writing in the margin places extra emphasis on the information. Be sure to draw an arrow from the margin to the place in the text that the word, concept, or date appears. By writing this information in the text, it is easy to review at a later time and the act of writing it will help you remember the information, too.

---

5. Raphael & Au, 2005

6. Peverly et al., 2007; Raphael & Au, 2005; Terry, 2006; Titsworth & Kiewra, 2004; Williams & Eggert, 2002

Test-taking strategies for multiple-choice questions

As we shared earlier, the TEAS is a multiple-choice test. Learning specific test-taking strategies for a multiple choice test can improve your overall test performance by helping you eliminate incorrect response choices[7]. For example, if a question has four potential options (i.e., A, B, C, or D), you automatically have a 25% chance of selecting the correct answer. However, if you can eliminate one or more of the four response options, you have a better chance of selecting the correct answer.

Tips

· **Rule out wrong answers.** By using your existing knowledge, you might be able to identify an incorrect answer. Eliminate incorrect answers and focus on the remaining choices.

· **Cover up the choices and answer the question.** The choices might make you second-guess yourself. If you know the answer without looking at the choices, then choose the option closest to your answer and don't second-guess yourself by reading the distractors.

· **Recognize opposite response options.** Often, if you find two opposite response choices, one is probably correct.

· **Look for absolute words.** Look for words that tend to make statements incorrect (e.g., always, never, all, only, must, and will). Statements using absolute or definite words tend to be incorrect because they do not apply in all situations.

· **Make educated guesses.** If you can't decide which response choice is best, make an educated guess.

· **Work backward.** Sometimes, you might have more success in answering a question by looking at the options first and working backward. This technique is especially useful in math questions.

Improving your score

Did you achieve the score you wanted on the test? If so, congratulations! If not, re-evaluate your study and test-taking strategies. Which strategies worked? Which ones did not? Research suggests that the more active strategies you implement into your studying, the better your performance in that class[8]. Consider the following hands-on strategy tips if you think you need to change your study habits or need suggestions for improving your test score.

Tips

· **Implement new study strategies immediately.** If you are unhappy with your results, try a new study strategy and implement it right away.

· **Join a study group.** If you normally study alone, consider studying with others.

· **If you are in a study group, assess how the group uses the study time.** Is the group mainly on task, or are there a lot of side conversations?

· **Spend individual time studying.** Plan to spend some time studying by yourself. After all, you are not taking the test as a group.

· **Seek other sources, including non-text sources.** If you need greater insight into a specific topic, seek out additional online educational sites, a tutor, or texts to enhance your learning.

· **Ask yourself questions that reinforce your learning.** For example, "If I had to teach this concept to another individual, how would I explain it?" or "If someone asked me to summarize this concept, what would I say?"

· **Consult an academic advisor if you are experiencing test anxiety and cannot manage it.** If you are feeling a lot of anxiety before and during a test, an advisor might be able to provide you with some extra tips for overcoming the anxiety.

· **Re-evaluate your work and extracurricular schedule.** If you are working or have extracurricular activities, consider reducing your hours at these activities so that you can spend more time studying. Alternatively, try changing the timing of your activities so that you study when you are most alert.

---

7. Paris et al., 1991

8. Gettinger & Seibert, 2002

Reading

The objectives for the Reading section of the TEAS are organized in three categories.

Key ideas and details (R.1) *22 questions*

R.1.1. Summarize a complex text.
R.1.2. Infer the logical conclusion from a reading selection.
R.1.3. Identify the topic, main idea, and supporting details.
R.1.4. Follow a given set of directions.
R.1.5. Identify specific information from a printed communication.
R.1.6. Identify information from a graphic representation of information.
R.1.7. Recognize events in a sequence.

Craft and structure (R.2) *14 questions*

R.2.1. Distinguish between fact and opinion, biases, and stereotypes.
R.2.2. Recognize the structure of texts in various formats.
R.2.3. Interpret the meaning of words and phrases using context.
R.2.4. Determine the denotative meaning of words.
R.2.5. Evaluate the author's purpose in a given text.
R.2.6. Evaluate the author's point of view in a given text.
R.2.7. Use text features.

Integration of knowledge and ideas (R.3) *11 questions*

R.3.1. Identify primary sources in various media.
R.3.2. Use evidence from text to make predictions and inferences, and draw conclusions about a piece of writing.
R.3.3. Compare and contrast themes from print and other sources.
R.3.4. Evaluate an argument and its specific claims.
R.3.5. Evaluate and integrate data from multiple sources in various formats, including media.

Remember, there are 47 scored Reading items on the TEAS. These are divided as shown. In addition, there will be six unscored pretest items that can be in any of these categories.

The Reading section of the TEAS will include a number of reading passages or other sources for which more than one question will be posed. In fact, as many as seven questions can be asked based on a single reading passage. You'll need to read those sources and then refer back to them to answer the questions. The quiz at the end of this section will give you a good idea of the number and types of sources you will encounter and the questions that will accompany those sources.

R.1.1 *Summarize a complex text.*

Text comprehension is a vital part of reading, and the ability to summarize a complex text is a foundational demonstration of one's comprehension. In order to comprehend, you must identify the topic, or subject, of the passage or text. The topic is a noun or noun phrase that encapsulates the subject matter of the writing. Examples of topics include: arteries, acid, alleles, mammals, and recycling. Once you have identified the topic of a text, you can easily identify the purpose for the reading and answer, "What am I reading about?" and "What is important to know about it?" For clarification, the author will include key points, or supporting details, that systematically show and support the point the author is trying to make. For questions on this TEAS task, you'll need to identify topics and key points and use that knowledge to summarize complex texts.

Because the topic is the general subject of a sentence, it helps to practice asking the following question about the topic sentence: "What am I reading about?" Ask yourself that question about the following topic sentence.

> Viruses are spread in a number of ways.

The box below shows how the controlling idea can be retrieved from asking the question above.

Question	Topic
What am I reading about?	viruses

Next, the reader must ask the second question: "What is important to know about it?"

Question	Controlling idea
What is important to know about it?	spread in a number of ways

Once a reader has identified the topic, it is essential to be able to identify and rephrase the key points. A key question to ask oneself is, "How do these points illustrate the topic sentence?"

> Viruses are spread in a number of ways. These are typically categorized as contact or non-contact modes of transmission. Contact modes include: droplet spray, when the virus drops, as a result of coughing or sneezing, into or onto exposed mucus membranes; indirect transmission, when the virus is shared through an object or surface; and direct transmission, when the virus is shared through direct person-to-person contact. Non-contact spread of viruses can occur through airborne aerosols, when the virus diffuses though the air into the lungs.

The key ideas in the above passage illustrate the topic sentence by describing how the spread of viruses is categorized and defining four modes of transmission.

This objective includes, but is not limited to, the following examples of knowledge, skills, and abilities.

- *Identify the topic.*
- *Identify key points.*
- *Rephrase key points.*

Key terms

controlling idea. The main idea of a text.

key ideas. Ideas that support controlling idea.

rephrase. Explain an idea in different words.

Next, a reader must be able to use the hints in the details to synthesize the key points in rephrasing ideas. The first step in rephrasing is to analyze (break down) the key ideas.

Key idea	Analysis (breakdown)
droplet, when the virus drops, as a result of coughing or sneezing, into or onto exposed mucus membranes	contact; airborne; drops; mucus membranes
indirect transmission, when the virus is shared through an object or surface	contact; object/surface
direct transmission, when the virus is shared through direct person-to-person contact	contact; person-to-person
aerosol, when the virus diffuses though the air into the lungs	non-contact; diffuse; airborne; lungs

Finally, it is time to rephrase the key ideas for understanding the main idea. Evaluate the similarities and differences in the key ideas and rephrase. Below is one rephrasing of the example passage.

There are multiple modes of virus transmission and these are categorized by whether or not the person contracting the virus came into contact with bodily fluids from an infected person.

R.1.1 Practice problems

Read the following passage. Then, answer the questions.

Choosing a hobby has multiple positive effects on a person. One positive effect is the alleviation of stress. There is a chemical change that occurs in a body when a person engages in an entertaining endeavor. The second positive effect is the building of confidence. Practicing and engaging in a hobby allows a person to feel successful by being good at something. Ultimately, when one becomes successful, self-esteem increases. The third reason to choose a hobby is the opportunity to meet new, interesting people. Most hobbies have many people already taking part. It is easy, especially with social media, to find people with the same interests. Finding common ground will bring people together in diverse social formats and allow for stimulating engagement opportunities. These three positive results of getting a hobby should entice anyone to go out and find something interesting to do.

1. Which of the following titles best synthesizes the key ideas?

   A. Find a hobby, find social media

   B. Find a hobby, find affirmative results

   C. Find a hobby, find peace

   D. Find a hobby, find a friend

2. Which of the following is the topic of the passage?

   A. Choosing a hobby

   B. Positive effects of a hobby

   C. Chemical change

   D. Social media

3. What is a logical rephrasing of the key ideas?

R.1.2 *Infer the logical conclusion from a reading selection.*

Whether you are reading an informational text, procedure, news article, or story, having the ability to infer logical conclusions based on what you've read is a true test of your comprehension. All writing has some level of suggestion because various readers' experiences bring diverse relatability to a passage. But key terms and descriptions provide structure for common understanding. To prepare for this TEAS task, look for key terms—including those providing information about events—that should lead you to a particular conclusion. Practice asking yourself, "What can I infer based on what I've just read?"

Critical readers make sense of passages by evaluating the information provided. Strong readers use individual experiences, in addition to the text, to construct meaning. In order to use the text, the reader must observe facts, delineate arguments, and discern valid information provided by the author. Then, the reader must combine what the author has provided with individual experiences to draw inference from the selection. Inference is reading between the lines of what is stated. In other words, it is applying logic (experience) to facts and evidence coupled with recognizing the context clues provided.

Identifying key terms is critical to understanding the context of a given passage. Key terms include those that provide sequence or chronology, descriptive words and phrases, and words that convey value judgments and opinion. These key terms can provide both explicit information and the implicit information that allows the reader to make inferences. Take this example:

> There **was a time** when I would have put up with his dismissive behavior, but those days, I'm **happy** to report, are long gone.

We can infer from the passage that the writer was previously a more passive person based on the key terms related to chronology, and we can infer that the writer prefers his or her current attitude based on the key term related to a value judgment. We can conclude from these inferences that the writer had a confrontation with the person mentioned in this sentence.

Many readers assume that making an inference and drawing a conclusion are the same. Each activity demands that a reader fill in some blanks. However, there is a subtle difference between the two. An inference suggests an idea by details and evidence in a passage. A conclusion asks the reader to analyze and make a decision based on predictions, details, evidence, and results. Below is an example of using inferences (clues in bold) to **draw a conclusion**.

> The fisherman stood on the banks of the lake, eyeing the **sluggish fish** come close to his line but never bite. **As he waited for the sun to go behind the mountain,** the **sweat stains** on his shirt grew in diameter.

Conclusion: The man is fishing in the midafternoon and it is too hot for the fish to bite. It is safe to predict that he thinks he will have better success in the evening.

This objective includes, but is not limited to, the following examples of knowledge, skills, and abilities.

- *Use inferences based on information given.*
- *Identify key terms justifying the events selected.*
- *Assemble events identified and associated with the inferred information to draw a conclusion.*

Key terms

conclusion. A deduction made by a reader about an unstated outcome from a reading passage.

explicit. Clearly stated.

implication. Something not clearly stated.

inference. A conclusion reached by critical thinking.

logic. The framework of reasoning used to understand ideas.

R.1.2 Practice problems

Read the following passage. Then, answer the questions.

Every 2 weeks, when Ray arrives home, the first thing he does is put his bag of muddy, oily clothes on top of the industrial washing machine he and Lori purchased last year. Lori insisted they buy the wash machine so she could do his laundry separate from the family's daily wash. After he unpacks from his 2 weeks away, he showers in order to be refreshed for his family. Then, he plays some games in the yard with the kids. Finally, the family goes to dinner so Lori does not have to make a dinner and do laundry.

1. Which of the following is Ray's job?

   A. Farrier

   B. Teacher

   C. Rig worker

   D. Electrician

2. Which of the following phrases helps the reader assemble the events in this passage?

   A. the first thing

   B. on top of

   C. separate from

   D. with the kids

3. What conclusions can be drawn about Ray and Lori's relationship?

R.1.3 *Identify the topic, main idea, and supporting details.*

This objective includes, but is not limited to, the following examples of knowledge, skills, and abilities.

• *Determine the topic.*

• *Determine the main idea.*

• *Explain how supporting details support the main idea.*

Key terms

comprehension. Ability to understand.

delineate. Describe precisely.

evidence. Proof to support an idea.

identify. Distinguish a particular idea.

imply. Indicate an idea subtly without specifically stating it.

irrelevant. Not applicable to the idea.

reason. A basis or fact to support an idea.

relevant. Connected to the idea being discussed.

topic. Subject of a text.

Critical reading demands that you become a selective consumer of text. Just like comparing essential vs. nonessential ingredients when shopping for healthy foods, a reader must identify the topic and author's main idea, and then delineate the author's key points that support the topic. Ultimately, the reader must demonstrate comprehension of a text by explaining how supporting details clarify the main idea. To succeed on this TEAS task, practice asking yourself, "What's the topic and what's the author's main idea about that topic?" Then examine the supporting details provided by the author and how they relate to the main idea.

To prepare for this section of the exam, be aware of the placement of the topic sentence and practice identifying the points an author makes. Read the passage in order to identify the main idea. Then locate the sentence(s) that emphasize, elaborate, or clarify this information. The topic answers the question, "Who or what is this paragraph about?" The topic should appear near the beginning of the paragraph and include the main idea. A topic sentence must not be too specific or too general.

> The lack of basic reading skills influences the low success rate of adolescent readers.

Notice that this topic sentence is not too specific (does not discuss the skills), nor too general (leaving out adolescent readers).

Supporting details develop—through explanation, elaboration, or clarification—the idea portrayed in the topic sentence. One way to identify the supporting or key ideas is to ask the following of the topic sentence: who, what, when, where, why, and how?

In the example below, the combination of key ideas clarifies which adolescent readers (LD and ADD/ADHD) and support the effects of the lack of reading skills.

> **Learning-disabled (LD) and attention deficit disorder/attention deficit hyperactivity disorder (ADD/ADHD) teenagers** suffer from lack of developed reading skills, and a high percentage of these young adult readers need assistance in transitioning into quality and complex level literacy. **Without the skills to scaffold their reading, students will lack the desire to read, or for that matter, adopt and practice the literacy demanded in career or college as mandated by the Common Core State Standards.**

Just as important as identifying the key ideas is discerning between relevant and irrelevant details. The relevant ideas relate back to the topic sentence. Irrelevant statements are unrelated and, at times, random. The bolded statements in the example below are irrelevant to the topic of the effects of exercise on physical and mental health.

> Exercise is good for anyone's physical and mental well-being. Statistics prove that aerobic exercise is good for the heart and muscles, ultimately enhancing and invigorating one's mind. **I used to ski race, but now I hike with my dogs for aerobic purposes.** In addition to aerobic exercise is the strength training component. In order to maintain bone density, increasing muscle mass is essential. **My mother continues to lift small weights to maintain her muscle mass.** Choosing to maintain a healthy lifestyle will benefit one's longevity.

R.1.3 Practice problems

Read the following passage. Then, answer the questions.

There is much more to training a horse than giving it a name. The most important element in training is time. A trainer must be prepared to spend time every day with the equine. Ground and body work must be implemented every session. The ground work can consist of backing strategies, while the body work can include ropes routinely wrapping different parts of the horse's body. All in all, the name is important but it is only the beginning.

1. What does the topic sentence imply?

2. How does the summary sentence support the topic sentence?

3. Reread the passage. Which of the following statements is a supporting detail?

   A. All in all, the name is important but it is only the beginning.

   B. There is much more to training a horse than giving it a name.

   C. Ground and body work must be implemented every session.

   D. Training a horse is time consuming.

Read the following excerpt from an online news feed. Then, answer the question.

Due to the high levels of rain this spring, residents of Garfield Street are warned to prepare for flooding by collecting and storing valuables, and finding shelter for pets. Valuables include photo albums, letters, and financial records. Consider purchasing a rental space or contacting community members for garage space. In order to protect your pets, consider calling the local veterinarian or animal shelter for short-term care.

4. Which of the following statements is the topic sentence?

   A. Consider purchasing a rental space or contacting community members for garage space.

   B. Valuables include photo albums, letters, and financial records.

   C. In order to protect your pets, consider calling the local veterinarian or animal shelter for short-term care.

   D. Due to the high levels of rain this spring, residents of Garfield Street are warned to prepare for flooding by collecting and storing valuables, and finding shelter for pets.

R.1.4 *Follow a given set of directions.*

This objective includes, but is not limited to, the following examples of knowledge, skills, and abilities.

- *Recognize the relationship among steps in a procedure.*
- *Identify key terms that signify order.*
- *Follow question directives, such as "choose all that apply."*

Readers and writers encounter procedural documents in all areas of learning. For example, engineering students read procedural programs, nursing students read pain management procedures, and chemistry students read laboratory procedures. In daily life, all readers must be prepared to read and follow procedures. Procedures can be found in any text, from recipes to vehicle manuals. This genre of sequential information offers readers the ability to safely, efficiently, and effectively complete activities. For the TEAS, you'll need to demonstrate the ability to follow directions by identifying important terms and recognizing the relationships among delineated tasks.

Language features and structures are specific to the organization and comprehension of procedural texts. The language features include signal words that assist the reader in recognizing the relationship among steps, and simple, objective language. Objective language is impartial, non-judgmental, non-personal, and non-emotional.

Procedural signal words

first	second	next	last
then	finally	while	before
second	now	when	after

Once a reader identifies all features of the procedure, it is important to follow all directions. Directions are very specific, using language that tells how to accomplish the steps. Some examples of these are listed in the box below.

From left to right	Carefully and with
After it has set	Choose all that apply
While the … complete steps	From top to bottom

The most common types of procedural texts include steps in an activity and steps in operating a system or object. The highest-occurring components of procedural writing include headings/subheading; numbering/alphabetizing steps; and charts, diagrams, and photographs for clarification of steps.

Key terms

edit. Correct errors in a piece of writing.

procedure. Process for writing, editing, and revision.

revision. Rewriting a piece of text.

sequence. Logical order in writing.

R.1.4 Practice problems

Read the passage below and answer the first two questions that follow.

*1. **Prewriting**. First, a writer must find the topic or idea by surveying day-to-day experiences, childhood memories, class topics, etc. Then a writer must build upon an idea by freewriting. Finally, the writer must plan and structure (outline) the writing. The structure must be relevant to the writing prompt or genre.*

*2. **Draft**. This step is very similar to freewriting in that the author does not worry about conventions (spelling and grammar). However, the author will use the outline as a guide. This is the first draft and offers much more freedom to the writer.*

*3. **Revision**. This third step includes four components. It is the step that makes the writing "beefy." First, the author must look at the draft and add information to clarify and enhance the text for the reader. Second, the author must rearrange the text so the flow, pace, and sequence of the events are in logical order. Third, the author must remove any unnecessary information or description. Fourth, the author must identify weak information or description and replace with effective text.*

*4. **Editing**. The text has been reviewed and revised for big ideas. Now it is time to fine-tune the piece of writing. This is the time to check—carefully and diligently—the spelling and grammar. Most importantly, the author needs to make sure the text flows and keeps the reader engaged.*

*5. **Publishing**. This final step in the writing process is publishing the text. This can include posting for a class, printing an advertisement, or sending a finalized letter.*

1. Which of the following is not a step in the revision process?
   - A. Add information to the draft.
   - B. Rearrange the text.
   - C. Edit the sentences.
   - D. Remove unnecessary information.

2. Identify the correct order of the writing process.
   - A. Prewrite, draft, revise, edit, publish
   - B. Draft, prewrite, revise, edit, publish
   - C. Prewrite, revise, draft, edit, publish
   - D. Draft, edit, prewrite, revise, publish

3. List five opportunities to write procedural texts.

R.1.5 *Identify specific information from a printed communication.*

The Latin definition of communication is the root *communis*, meaning to make common, impart, inform, and share. Printed communication, such as memos, announcements, and advertisements fulfill this definition. Many types of printed communication join together people who have common interests, and share information amongst those that desire further detail. It is beneficial to understand how to discern relevant information and recognize the text structures of printed communication. The TEAS will test how well you can find the information you need from these types of communications.

A memo, though more informal that other printed communication, is usually concise and grammatically correct. The formal format results from the audience usually being internal (business staff members, school colleagues, etc.). Correct conventions are important because the information is usually business-oriented. See a sample memo and descriptions below.

Memorandum

To: Recipient(s)

From: Author of the memo and title

Date: Date memo is shared

Re: The subject of the memo

Introductory: Informs the readers of the specific context of the memo.

Each body section should start with a strong, concise statement (claim) that informs the reader of the important information. Readers only want the important information and nothing extra.

Concluding Section: Includes strong rephrased take-away information. This section can also include where to address any questions or concerns. There is no need to mention the author's name. The author is mentioned in the heading.

Printed public announcements

Memos are one way to get information to a group of people. Another efficient way is by posted announcements. One such printed communication is the public announcement. These come in various forms, but they have multiple basic elements. Public announcements inform the public about organizations, upcoming events, and services. The message must be short, the design simple and eye-pleasing, and the important information easily accessible. The content should include a link to information access, information about the supporting organizations, and supporting details. The supporting details should be in images and short phrases if possible.

See the example and descriptions.

This objective includes, but is not limited to, the following examples of knowledge, skills, and abilities.

- *Use printed communications (e.g., memos, posted announcements, classified ads).*
- *Find relevant information.*
- *Recognize various parts of printed communications.*

Key terms

blog. A website that is usually informal and independently run.

classified. A print advertisement selling or soliciting something.

exclamatory. With strong emotion.

forum. An online message board.

rhetorical. Used for effect only, not meaning.

memorandum. A written informal note usually used for business purposes.

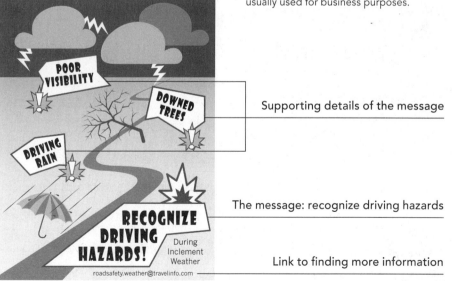

Supporting details of the message

The message: recognize driving hazards

Link to finding more information

Classified advertisements

The classified advertisement is generally a short, detailed text offering items and services. Print and online newspapers, magazines, blogs, and forums usually charge by the word or line. Therefore, a reader can find the following information within a very small space.

- A headline that engages the reader in seconds (can be a rhetorical question, bold statement, or exclamation)

- An item or service offered to the audience (mentions the benefits of the item or service)

- A call to action (includes how to get the item or service)

See this sample and description of an online classified advertisement.

Headline that attracts a specific audience	**Need outdoor pictures taken for that special event?**
Mentions benefits in order to attract a consumer	Choose your own setting, time, and subject. Choose your own time frame for development and packages.
Call to action tells consumer what to do next	Please email jerome@sunshinephotos.com or call 555-345-6758 and let the photos begin!

R.1.5 Practice problems

Read the following memo and answer the first question.

Memorandum
Superintendent's Office School District #6
To: *Teaching Staff*
From: *Dr. Billings, Superintendent*
Date: *May 18*
Re: *Summer Training Offerings*

The school district is offering three summer training sessions for those interested in making extra money and experiencing breakthrough academic strategies.

Title	Location	Dates	Lodging
It's All About the Verb	Simsville College, Room 106	July 8–10	Hillsboro Hotel
The Equation of a Lifetime	Simsville College, Room 106	July 15–17	Hillsboro Hotel
History is a Living Thing	Simsville College, Room 106	August 2–4	Hillsboro Hotel

Registration: *Click on the registration link and complete all questions.*
www.registrationtraining.org

Accommodations: *When making hotel reservations, please call 555-478-7272 and mention School District #6 block of rooms.*

Stipend information: *Please fill out the attached invoice and turn into the business office by August 13.*

1. Which of the following describes how an attendee can get reservations in the correct hotel?
   A. Email the hotel.
   B. Call the specified phone number.
   C. Fill out the voucher.
   D. Click on the registration link.

2. Which of the following identifies four features of a printed public announcement?
   A. Name of an item, message, supporting detail, a lot of color
   B. Organization, supporting detail, information link, correct spelling
   C. Organization, message, supporting detail, information link
   D. Images, message, supporting detail, information link

3. List three media in which classified advertisements are found.

R.1.6 *Identify information from a graphic representation of information.*

Many texts portray information through graphic representations. These pictorial images allow readers to comprehend important verbal and written ideas in accessible and succinct form. Most graphic representations include titles and subheads that summarize complex information. Graphics can also assist readers in selecting important information that might otherwise be missing by portraying the key parts that make up a whole. Graphic representations include bar, pie, and flow charts, graphs, maps, and illustrations. When you take the TEAS, you'll likely be tested on your knowledge of these tools and your ability to interpret the information they provide.

Graphic representations can illustrate diverse topics and designs, but common features include titles, subheads, keys/legends, and scales. Learning how to read maps, pictures, and graphs hones and replicates the skills needed to read information. One must be able to identify the features in graphic representations just as readers must identify elements when reading informational texts.

This objective includes, but is not limited to, the following examples of knowledge, skills, and abilities.

- *Read a graphic representation (e.g., map, pictograph).*
- *Identify relevant information.*
- *Recognize visuals, graphics, and figures within the text.*
- *Locate the important information from a graphic representation.*

Features of graphic representations

Maps come in many sizes and shapes, but most include the common elements of titles, legends, and scales. The title articulates the purpose of the map. The legend clarifies what each symbol, color, or shape represents. Lastly, the scale represents the distance between points.

The Tri-Park Campground figure provides an example of map features.

The features on the map tell readers that the length of the scale ruler is 1 kilometer. The legend combined with the title tells the reader that the map illustrates the location of the campgrounds. The features on the legend—interstate, highway, and construction—imply that the driver will be passing through construction on the way to the parks. This is a prime example of key pieces portrayed in a holistic picture.

Key terms

graphic. A diagram, graph, illustration, or other piece of artwork.

legend. Map feature that explains symbols and other elements.

representation. How something is expressed.

scale. Ratio of distance expressed to actual measurement.

Practice

Which of the following statements is accurate based on the map?

A. Park #3 is the southernmost park.
B. A driver would take I-50 westbound to reach these parks.
C. Park #1 has lakes on either side.
D. The drive from Park #2 to Park #3 is about 500 meters.

Rationale: Option A is correct because the compass indicates that the bottom of the map correlates with a southern direction, and Park #3 is below the other two parks. Option B is incorrect because I-50 is a north–south interstate. Option C is incorrect because both lakes represented in the map are south of Park #1. Option D is incorrect because the scale indicates that Park #2 and Park #3 are about 3 kilometers driving distance apart.

Pictorial representations come in many designs that depend on the purpose and content. Interpreting these involves many of the same skills required in reading informational writing. For example, the pictorial graph will include a combination of titles, subheads, summaries, descriptions, images representing ideas, content vocabulary, steps in a process, and data. Sometimes, this information will already be analyzed for the readers. But more likely, the representation requires a reader's understanding and analysis.

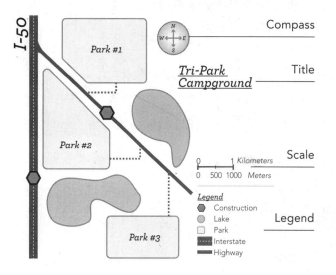

The following is an example of some of the features of pictorial representations.

Practice

Which of the following is indicated by this drawing?

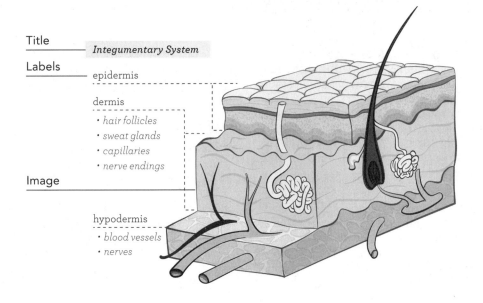

Title —————— *Integumentary System*

Labels —————— epidermis

dermis
· *hair follicles*
· *sweat glands*
· *capillaries*
· *nerve endings*

Image ——————

hypodermis
· *blood vessels*
· *nerves*

A. Nerve endings are part of the hypodermis.
B. The epidermis includes the dermis.
C. Hair follicles can be found in the dermis.
D. Nerves exist only in the hypodermis.

Rationale: Option C is correct because the drawing shows both textually and in the drawing that hair follicles originate in the dermis. Option A is not correct because nerve endings are shown in the dermis. Option B is not correct because the drawing indicates that the epidermis and dermis are distinct, coequal parts of the integumentary system. Option D is not correct because nerve endings can be found in the dermis.

R.1.6 Practice problems

Use the graphic representation to answer the following questions.

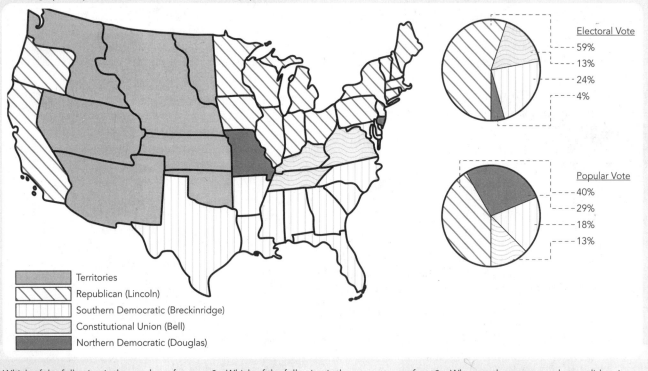

Electoral Vote
59%
13%
24%
4%

Popular Vote
40%
29%
18%
13%

Territories
Republican (Lincoln)
Southern Democratic (Breckinridge)
Constitutional Union (Bell)
Northern Democratic (Douglas)

1. Which of the following is the number of remaining territories in 1860?
   A. 10
   B. 7
   C. 5
   D. 11

2. Which of the following is the percentage of the electoral vote Douglas received?
   A. 24%
   B. 9%
   C. 4%
   D. 13%

3. Who was the most popular candidate in 1860? What was the spread between the most and second-most popular candidates?

R.1.7 *Recognize events in a sequence.*

Sequence refers to order and pattern, and recognizing sequence has powerful benefits, such as remembering information, understanding text, and analyzing information for comprehension. One thing to consider is the subtle difference between sequential and chronological ordering within text. *Sequential* refers to a fixed order in which there is a logical pattern. Pages in a book, for example, are sequential, as are steps in a process. *Chronological* refers to events in an order in which they happen and requires a time element. For this TEAS task, you'll need to understand these concepts and be able to interpret the words and phrases that create sequence.

In order to find meaning in text, it is crucial to understand how to find and order the events or ideas. Signal words assist a reader with fitting smaller parts of the text into a larger context.

Sequential order is signaled by words such as the following.

first	second	next	last
then	finally	while	before
second	now	when	after
at the beginning	prior to	afterward	subsequently

Below is an example of a passage with sequential order words bolded.

> Sue offered to help her friends prepare for the barbecue. **First,** she made a healthy salad. **Second,** she baked a carrot cake; and, **finally,** she picked up several bags of ice.

Due to the use of sequence signal words, there is no question the logical order of Sue's preparations.

Chronological signal words describe when one event occurs and ends, and when another event begins. Readers must be aware of these terms, which function as adverbs. They refer to when something happened, how often an event occurs, or for the length time an event occurs. The following is a list of adverbs that signal the above chronological events.

When	*How often*	*Length of time*
today	always	all year
yesterday	rarely	all season
later	often	all day
now	never	since
last year	seldom	one day

This objective includes, but is not limited to, the following examples of knowledge, skills, and abilities.

- *Understand the concept of sequence.*
- *Locate the words or phrases that indicate sequence of events (e.g., first, second, third).*
- *Identify language that indicates time (e.g., today, tomorrow).*

Key terms

chronological. In order by time.
sequential. Following a set order.

Below is an example of a passage with chronological order words bolded.

> **One day** while walking home from school, Tom found a rare rock. **When** he put it in his pocket, he turned empowered. **At first,** he used his new-found strength to play tricks on those that harassed him. He'd turned so bold **since** finding this ability. **Often,** he did not know when he had gone too far. **For a year,** he seemed to be making many new friends; but **after a while,** he realized they were just fearful of being on his bad side, and he became very lonely. **Finally,** he threw away the rock and became the friend he was meant to be.

Chronological signal words are essential in assisting readers with keeping track of occasions in narratives and informational texts, such as passages relaying historical events. In the above passage, the author mentions what Tom did upon finding the rock. Then the reader experiences a year of events until Tom chooses to throw away the rock. Without time signals, the reader could get very confused.

R.1.7 Practice problems

Read the following passage and answer the first two questions.

This morning was senseless. First, I forgot to set my alarm clock, so I awoke to the sound of the mail coming through the slot in my door. Instantly, I threw on some clothes and bolted for the door. I rarely have to hurry this fast, so I left without a cup of coffee. After what seemed like forever, I arrived at work and everyone was entering the front of the office building. Since this crazy experience, I have made it a point to set my alarm clock. Looking back, it wasn't mail coming through the slot in the door. Instead, I think it was ice falling on the porch.

1. Choose the statement that is out of sequence.

   A. Instantly, I threw on some clothes and bolted for the door.

   B. After what seemed like forever, I arrived at work and everyone was entering the front of the office building.

   C. Since this crazy experience, I have made it a point to set my alarm clock.

   D. Looking back, it wasn't the mail coming through the slot in the door.

2. Which of the words or phrases from the passage indicates sequence?

   A. This morning

   B. First

   C. Instantly

   D. like forever

3. Which of the following is the correct sequence of events for the scientific method?

   1. Ask a question to begin the process.

   2. Ultimately, accept or decline the hypothesis.

   3. Propose a hypothesis as a result of research into the topic.

   4. In order to analyze data, perform the experiment

   5. Analyze the data.

   6. Conduct background research on the identified question.

   A. 1, 2, 4, 6, 3, 5

   B. 1, 6, 3, 4, 5, 2

   C. 2, 3, 6, 5, 1, 4

   D. 3, 6, 2, 1, 5, 4

Practice problem answers

R.1.1

1. Option B is correct. It synthesizes all three key ideas. Option A only reflects the clarification of the third reason. Option C summarizes the first point. Option D only reflects the third key idea.
2. Option A is correct. Choosing a hobby is the topic of the passage. Option B is the main idea of the topic sentence. Option C is detail for the first key idea. Option D is detail for the third key idea.
3. Rationale: Rephrasing of key ideas could include the following.
   - Hobbies help reduce stress.
   - Hobbies can build confidence.
   - Hobbies can help build your social network.

R.1.2

1. Option C is correct. Clues such as every two weeks, muddy, and oily combined with a reader's knowledge of oil rigs imply Ray's job. Farrier is incorrect because there is no implication of Ray working with horses. Teacher is incorrect because there is no hint that he teaches. Electrician is incorrect due to lack of hints toward electrical work.
2. Option A is correct because this phrase provides a sequence context for the actions that Ray takes when he arrives home. The first thing he does is to put his clothes on top of the washing machine. The other options do not provide any information that would allow the reader to assemble the events in the passage.
3. Ray respects Lori and the amount of work she has to do when he gets home. This is implied when the passage states, "Finally, the family goes to dinner so Lori does not have to make a dinner and do laundry."

R.1.3

1. The phrase "…much more to training…" tells the reader there is more information coming in the paragraph. In addition, the author implies that naming a horse is also important by using the comparison ("…more to training a horse than giving it a name").
2. The transition into the summary sentence (all in all) shows the passage is concluding. Plus, the remainder of the sentence reiterates that naming is important but that there is much more ("…only the beginning") to training.
3. Option C supports the topic sentence that there is more to training than naming the horse. Option A is the summary sentence. Option B is the topic sentence. Option D is a generalization made from the reading.
4. Option D is the topic sentence. It is not too general (just mentioning that residents are to prepare for flooding), yet it is not too specific (fully explaining how residents are to collect and store valuables and find shelter for pets). Collecting and storing valuables and finding shelter for pets are the main ideas mentioned in the topic sentence. What valuables can consist of (photo albums, letters, financial records) and types of storage (rental or garage space), and calling a local veterinarian or shelter all elaborate upon the main ideas in the topic sentence. Option A is supporting detail for storing valuables. Option B is supporting detail that illustrates examples of valuables. Option C is supporting detail on how to find shelter for pets.

R.1.4

1. Option C is correct because it is an editing step; plus, this choice is not mentioned in the revision section with a sequential signal word. Option A is the first revision step. Option B is the second revision step. Option D is the third revision step.
2. Option A is correct because the steps are numbered and match. The remaining choices are incorrect because they do not match the sequential numbering or the logical steps described in the process.
3. Answers could include recipes, scientific labs, creating a web page, or playing scales on musical instruments.

R.1.5

1. Option B is correct because the specific information is offered in the accommodations section. Option A is incorrect because an email is not offered under accommodations. Option C is incorrect because the voucher is for the stipend. Option D is incorrect because the link is for registration.
2. Option C is correct because these are the crucial features of an announcement. Option A is incorrect because use of color is nice, but not as important as the information link, message, supporting detail, and organization. Option B is incorrect because correct spelling is crucial in the publishing but is not a feature. Option D is incorrect because images are not essential.
3. Answers might include print and online newspapers, blogs, forums, and magazines.

R.1.6

1. Option B is correct. The legend shows that gray depicts territories.
2. Option C is correct because 4% is shown in the electoral vote pie chart on top and matches the pattern that represents Douglas. Options A and D match the incorrect percentages and patterns in the upper pie chart. Option B is the number of votes, not the percentage.
3. Lincoln was the most popular candidate, with 40% of the popular votes. Lincoln beat Douglas by an 11% spread. This is depicted on the lower pie chart.

R.1.7

1. Option C is correct. It is out of sequence because the signal phrase "Since this crazy experience…" hints at a closing statement.
   - Option A is incorrect because instantly is a clue to a reaction to the sound mentioned in statement 1.
   - Option B is incorrect because the adverb after tells the reader that an event occurred next in a sequence, and the only apparent event is the preparing and leaving for work.
   - Option D is incorrect because the author is looking back at the awakening sound, which is mentioned earlier in the passage.
2. Option B is correct because it indicates that the sequence starts with the author forgetting to check his or her alarm clock. While the other options provide some information regarding time, they don't contribute to our understanding of the sequence of these events.
3. Option B is correct because all the hints and signal words make the sequence apparent: "begin the process," "identified question," "as a result of research," "in order to analyze," "analyze," "ultimately."

R.2.1 *Distinguish between fact and opinion, biases, and stereotypes.*

One of the challenges readers often face is to evaluate a writer's point of view. In order to identify point of view, readers will find it helpful to discern between fact and opinion, biases, and stereotypes. An author's word choice will sometimes portray a tone or feeling toward their topic. Becoming aware of the tone, word choice, biases or stereotypes, and use of fact or opinion allows a reader to critically evaluate an author's point of view. This TEAS task will assess your ability to analyze these aspects of various pieces of writing.

Point of view

Point of view is the way an author considers the subject of the writing. There are several ways that readers can identify the point of view for the purposes of in-depth comprehension, challenging the author and the text, and viewing the subject through diverse lenses.

Tool	Reason
Read multiple texts on same subject.	Compare facts, opinions, biases and stereotypes.
Identify author's word choice.	Recognize tone (author's feeling of subject).
Conclude what is missing from a text.	Determine POV by omission.
Imagine author's side in a debate.	Evaluate the biases and stereotypes.

Facts and opinions

In order to identify a statement as fact or opinion, it is essential to understand that a fact can be proven true or false. The reader must decide whether the facts are reliable. On the flip side, opinions can have a basis in facts but depend upon an author's beliefs portrayed in the text. Opinions can be used to mislead or persuade a reader.

Fact	Opinion
At least 23% of all automobile collisions involve cell phones.	Texting while driving is done by ignorant people.

This objective includes, but is not limited to, the following examples of knowledge, skills, and abilities.

- *Recognize factual writing as supported by evidence.*
- *Recognize author's point of view in a text (fact, opinion, biases, stereotypes).*
- *Recognize author's tone.*
- *Define stereotype and bias.*
- *Compare and contrast fact and opinion.*

Key terms

assumption. Supposition of an unstated idea.

bias. Tendency toward a preconceived idea.

fact. Statement that can be proven.

opinion. Statement that cannot be proven.

point of view. Perspective.

stereotype. Simplified categorization of an idea or person based on convention.

tone. The author's voice and attitude toward the topic.

Stereotypes and biases

To counterbalance stereotypes and biases, a reader must understand that a stereotype is a biased belief about a person or group and does not recognize individual differences or social distinction. Stereotypes are influenced by parents, peers, social opinions, and the media. It is beneficial to understand that stereotypes can be positive and negative. Regardless, stereotypes have negative consequences, whereas a bias is a preferential viewpoint that often does not allow for impartial or objective discussion.

Stereotypes and biases are commonly incorrectly interchanged. The following are some differences that assist identification.

Stereotype	Bias
Writer remains nonemotional and uses general statements.	Writer uses emotionally charged word choice and figurative language.
Writer might have facts based upon researched biases and falsely supported assumptions.	Writer purposefully omits facts due to a usual lack of validation.

R.2.1 Practice problems

1. Which of the following is a factual statement?

   A. Obesity is caused by inappropriate eating habits.

   B. Obese people do not have willpower.

   C. One in three adolescents is obese.

   D. Obese people just need to lose weight.

2. Discuss how this stereotype is harmful: "Japanese people are incredible engineers."

Since the late 16th century, the public has had a strange fascination with arctic expeditions. These expeditions are launched for many ostensible reasons: to chart new territory, to conduct scientific research, to search for oil, or simply to have an adventure. Consider the many hardships and tragedies of these expeditions: Franklin's memorable disaster, Shackleton's famous wreck, or the more recent tragedy of the Vladimir Karamenov. Ask yourself: Is all this loss of life worthwhile? What real, tangible gains have been made from these expeditions? A few more marks and scribbles on our world maps? A few more frozen, useless islands that now possess explorers' names? The entire concept of the arctic expedition is folly. The subject, and, indeed, this entire area of the world, should be abandoned until such time as fully automated research ships can be sent into the polar wastes. Only then, when no human life is at risk, should these dangerous efforts resume. In the meantime, we should not look back at the early arctic explorers as heroes or legends. We should not honor them with statues, plaques, or lengthy entries in our history books. Rather, we should shake our heads at their foolishness, and transfer our admiration to people who have made real discoveries in other, more practical fields of knowledge.

3. Which of the following statements best aligns with the author's point of view?

   A. Franklin's arctic expedition is a memorable story.

   B. Arctic explorers' self-gratifying expeditions should be ignored.

   C. Adventure is an adequate reason to risk the hardships of arctic exploration.

   D. Human life should never be risked for scientific pursuits.

R.2.2 *Recognize the structure of texts in various formats.*

Reading and writing is a continual puzzle-building game that can fit in different ways for diverse purposes. As a reader, you must be able to recognize various modes and types of texts. On the other hand, writers must use a blend of modes and types of writing to fulfill specific purposes. Modes are defined as classifications of rhetorical writing, such as persuasive, expository, and narrative. Types of writing are the texts that fall under each mode. For example, some of the types of writing that make up expository writing are compare/contrast, procedure, and cause and effect. Some narrative structures are myths, biographies, short stories, poetry, and novels. For the TEAS, you'll need to identify and evaluate these modes and the structures they employ.

Persuasive/argumentative

The persuasive/argumentative mode of writing allows the author to convince the reader to believe something about a topic. The author usually attempts to convince the reader to feel, think, or behave a certain way. In persuasive texts, the reader can find facts, details, examples, and persuasive word choice in addition to a logical order of thought development. Introductory and parenthetical phrases are common places for readers to discern the persuasive language in texts. Persuasive language must be able to portray strong opinions.

Strong opinion signal words and phrases

in the first place	without a doubt	undoubtedly	unquestionably
it is my belief that	all that to the side	from my point of view	I question whether

The facts, details, and examples are usually in a logical sequence following a claim. The claim, or topic sentence, proclaims the main focus of a paragraph and supports the main idea or thesis of the text. The reason answers *why* to any claim. The evidence *shows*—with the use of facts, details, or examples—what the claim *looks* like. In other words, it backs up the claim by proving it. A counterclaim is the opposition's reason against the author's claim, and a writer may anticipate and refute counterclaims. The analysis explains *how* the evidence is supporting the claim and wraps up the paragraph. Typically, persuasive texts follow a logical order of weakest argument to strongest argument.

Examples of claim, reasons, evidence, and analysis

Claim: "Dad, I deserve to have a new laptop for college."

Reason: "Dad, I graduated high school with very good grades."

Evidence: The transcript shows four As, two Bs, and two Cs.

Counterclaim: "Son, you have not earned a new laptop yet…"

Reason: "…because you have not yet received your first semester college grades."

Evidence: The college states that a 3.0 GPA is sufficient to keep scholarships.

Analysis: "The college expectations are what your mother and I are holding you accountable to keep. If you get a 3.0 GPA, we will buy the laptop for you."

This objective includes, but is not limited to, the following examples of knowledge, skills, and abilities.

- *Know the modes (e.g., persuasive, expository, narrative).*
- *Identify compare and contrast.*
- *State cause and effect.*
- *Recognize problem solution.*

Key terms

anecdote. A short story that illustrates a concept but is not the main idea.

argumentative. A contentious tone.

modes. Forms of writing.

persuasive. Intending to make the reader believe an idea.

rhetoric. The use of elements of language.

structures. Ways of logically organizing ideas.

Problem/solution

One common persuasive type of essay is the problem/solution structure. This structure includes the following: introduction of the problem being addressed, a description of the problem, a plausible solution to the problem, and a closing that challenges the reader to take action. The format can change, but these features make up a problem/solution essay. The following box includes some signal words and phrases for problem/solution essays.

the problem	so that	for this reason	if... then...
because	this led to	a solution	one reason for

Expository

In the expository mode of writing, the author informs, explains, or tells *how to*. In contrast to persuasive writing, expository writing does not include opinions but only uses facts and examples. As such, many expository texts use a structure similar to the claim, evidence, and analysis of the persuasive mode. Similar to persuasive, expository uses a logical order of least to most important, most to least important, or a detailed step-by-step process.

As in any writing, expository texts have very specific signal words and phrases. The boxes below illustrate some of those important signals.

Cause and effect

The CAUSE is *why* something happens.

The EFFECT is *what happened*.

due to	consequently	as a result of	if... then...
was responsible for	as might be expected	made possible by	since

Compare/contrast

To COMPARE is to find similarities.

To CONTRAST is to identify differences.

on the contrary	similarly	have in common	in spite of
in like manner	compared to	in the same way	as well as

Procedure

first	next	then	in closing
to begin with	accordingly	last	to finish

Narrative

The narrative mode has several purposes; authors can entertain, inform, and challenge their readers through diverse structures. Narratives tell stories with sensory details that assist the readers in experiencing events. Whether in poetry, anecdotes, or short stories, narratives use chronological order (beginning to end or end to beginning). Yet, many authors use narrative devices that foreshadow or flash back and create images in readers' minds.

The following is a list of signal words and phrases that assist readers in following the order of events (time and sequential) in narrative writing.

abruptly	after a few days	gradually	instantly
from this point	this instant	until now	sporadically
on the next occasion	not long ago	previously	recently

R.2.2 Practice problems

Debra –

I just heard about the new executive opening. It seems a little unusual to add new people there, especially when some of the other departments need staff.

All that to the side, I think you should consider Alex Jones from Accounting. I think his skills are wasted at his current job; he would make an excellent manager. He's done everything we asked him to, and more. Everyone down here likes him, and I can't imagine him doing anything to disappoint you – or the company, for that matter. Just call him up for an interview, and I think you'll see what I mean.

Also, we're getting Chinese food delivered later, so give any menu requests to Andy.

Regards,

Hal

1. Which of the following identifies the mode of the passage?

   A. Expository

   B. Persuasive/argumentative

   C. Narrative

   D. Descriptive

Read the following passage and complete the next question.

Even though Arizona and Rhode Island are both states of the U.S., they are strikingly different in many ways. For example, the physical size of each state differs. Arizona is large, having an area of 114,000 square miles; _____ , Rhode Island is only a tenth the size, having an area of only 1, 214 square miles. Another difference is in the size of the population of each state. Arizona has 4 million people living in it, but Rhode Island has less than 1 million. Also, the two states differ in the kids of natural environments that each has. For example, Arizona is a very dry state, consisting of large desert areas that do not receive much rainfall every year. On the flip side, Rhode Island is located in a temperate zone and receives an average of 44 inches of rain per year. [1]

2. Which of the following is the best signal word or phrase to fill in the blank?

   A. in like manner

   B. consequently

   C. in comparison

   D. in spite of

3. Describe the difference between reason and evidence.

_____

1. Adapted from Walters, F. Scott. "Comparison and Contrast Paragraphs. http://lrs.ed.uiuc.edu, 2000

R.2.3 *Interpret the meaning of words and phrases using context.*

This objective includes, but is not limited to, the following examples of knowledge, skills, and abilities.

- *Identify the correct definition of a word.*
- *Identify a source to find vocabulary definitions.*
- *Distinguish between figurative and connotative meanings.*
- *Recognize the cumulative effect of specific word choice on meaning.*

Key terms

connotation. An implied meaning of a word or idea.

denotation. An explicitly stated meaning of a word or idea.

figurative. By a figure of speech, usually a metaphor.

Reading comprehension is a difficult practice made more difficult by the multiple meanings of words. In order to be a successful reader, you must adeptly identify correct definitions, discern between diverse meanings, and distinguish between figurative and connotative word meaning. The TEAS will test your ability to skillfully employ these strategies and to evaluate the impact of an author's use of vocabulary in text.

Identify the correct definition of a word

Comprehending text is easier said than done. It involves multiple skills, one of which is identifying a correct definition of a word. In order to accomplish this task, first find meaning in context. The context is the text preceding or following a specific word. Several types of context clues provide hints to the meaning of the specific word.

Root words and affixes

A root is the base of a word (for example, fract) and can have a prefix or suffix (-tion) added to make meaning. In this instance, fract means to break and the suffix –tion means the act of. So the meaning of fraction, the act of breaking, becomes clear.

Contrasting signal phrases

> *Distinct from other poisons,* venom is produced and delivered by an animal.

In this example, the signal phrase provides the clue that a venom is a specific type of poison.

Definition

> Environmental poisons, *or those found in the water or air,* often have insidious effects.

In this example, the definition is provided as a restatement of the phrase.

Example or illustration

> Hydrocarbons, *such as kerosene and gasoline,* often have poisonous effects.

In this sentence, the examples given provide a hint as to the definition of a hydrocarbon.

Distinguishing between figurative and connotative meanings

Many authors employ creative ways to state ideas and make unfamiliar settings and objects more accessible to the reader. If a reader becomes aware of common figurative devices, then the text will be more manageable and comprehensible.

Figurative Device	Definition	Example
Metaphor	Comparison between unlike things without using like or as	The teacher **is** a lion.
Simile	Comparison between unlike things using like or as	The teacher is **like** a lion.
Personification	Giving human attributes to something nonhuman	The leaves **danced** in the wind.

Comprehension of a text can depend upon a reader's ability to infer the meaning of the word by reading between the author's lines. In addition to assisting comprehension, authors can influence the emotional effect upon a reader. One's experiences will determine the positive and negative connotations of a word. Ultimately, the tone (author's feeling toward the subject) affects the mood (the reader's feeling elicited from the text).

For example, each of the following words is very similar, yet experiences and use portray diverse meanings.

Word	Connotation
childlike	immature
youthful	lively, energetic

After using connotations and identifying roots and affixes, a reader might still use a dictionary, thesaurus, or other source to compare words and their meanings.

Book	Online
Dictionary	http://www.merriam-webster.com (online dictionary)
Thesaurus	http://www.visuwords.com (online graphical dictionary)
	http://graphwords.com (online visual thesaurus)

R.2.3 Practice problems

The ship ran aground on a great slab of ice. It had smashed its way almost to the Arctic Circle, but could press no farther. It made a terrible grating sound as it slid up onto the ice: it was the sound of absolute finality. We knew we could not break free. We settled down to wait; we had no choice. We ran the ship's engines to produce heat, and whiled away the days with card games and old magazines. But days turned into weeks, and soon the reserves were low. We had neither the fuel nor the food to keep this up indefinitely. On the third week, the captain made his decision: we loaded up the sled dogs and set out across the ice. We were apprehensive about leaving the ship, but we also knew that we could not stay. Every man – even those who professed no religion – prayed like a saint as we rode our sleds off into the gray distance.

1. Which of the following identifies the mood of the passage?

   A. Adventurous

   B. Excited

   C. Nervous

   D. Scared

We should shake our heads at explorers' foolishness, and transfer our admiration to people who have made real discoveries in other, more practical fields of knowledge.

2. Which of the following words from the sentence has a negative connotation?

   A. Foolishness

   B. Practical

   C. Real

   D. Admiration

It is a fact that a large number of small businesses fail because the owner hasn't enough capital to tide him over slack periods and emergencies; that is, it takes a certain amount of working money to keep a business going.

3. Which of the following is the meaning of capital in the passage?

   A. An exchange made to keep a business lucrative

   B. Money allotted for specific purposes

   C. The center of a town, state, nation

   D. A certain amount of working money to keep a business going

R.2.4 *Determine the denotative meaning of words.*

This objective includes, but is not limited to, the following examples of knowledge, skills, and abilities.

- *Identify the correct definition of a word.*
- *Identify a source to find vocabulary definitions.*

Key terms

context. Nearby text that influences understanding.

guide words. Words in a dictionary that help readers locate words.

parts of speech. Basic types of words in English.

word origin. How a word came to its current use and meaning.

Determining the meanings of words is one of the first and most basic skills in learning to read and comprehend text. Words have two levels of meaning: denotative and connotative. The denotative meaning of a word is its dictionary definition. The connotative meaning of a word is more complex, and is a combination of the word's definition and its suggested meaning based on context and emotions or associations evoked by a word. For the purposes of this TEAS task, we will focus on the *denotative* meaning of words and strategies for locating denotative word meanings.

Perhaps the easiest and most traditional way to find a word's meaning is to look up the word in a dictionary. There are several reliable and well-known dictionaries; the Merriam-Webster Dictionary and the Oxford English Dictionary are two you have probably seen in libraries, classrooms, and offices. These dictionaries are usually large books that require you to know little about a word prior to finding its meaning.

It is helpful to know how a word is spelled, or at least the first several letters of the word. This will not be a problem if you are looking up a word found in a text. However, if you have only heard the word and have not seen it in a printed text, you might have to guess about how it is spelled. Once you know the first several letters of a word, you should be able to locate it in the dictionary using guide words. Guide words appear at the top of each page of a dictionary and show readers the first and last words that appear on that page. You will need to search for the two guide words that would come before and after the word you are looking up. For example, to find the word "establish," a page with guide words "each" and "eclectic" would not include the word, but a page with guide words "escalator" and "evolve" would include the word.

Most dictionaries include a standard set of information intended to help a reader understand its meaning. Dictionaries usually include a word's part of speech, which refers to how the word functions within a sentence. Noun, verb, adjective, and adverb are common parts of speech. They are often abbreviated in dictionaries in the following ways.

Noun: *n.*

Verb: *v.*

Adjective: *adj.*

Adverb: *adv.*

If a word has multiple meanings, dictionaries will include a numbered list of meanings, usually followed by sentences that demonstrate the word being used with each meaning. Some dictionaries even include a word's origin, which can help readers make associations or connections with other words they might know.

Finding denotative word meanings has become easier due to technological advances. With a smartphone, tablet, or computer, simply type a word into a search box and quickly retrieve denotative word meanings. Both *Merriam-Webster* and *Oxford English Dictionary* offer online resources. Many of the basic principles followed in printed dictionaries also apply to online sources. Word meanings found online still typically include a part of speech and several possible definitions with examples to provide readers some context.

R.2.4 Practice problems

1. Which of the following sets of guide words would appear at the top of a printed dictionary page containing the word "aptitude"?

   A. anesthetize and anthology

   B. Appalachian and aviator

   C. allergic and apology

   D. area and army

2. Your friend came across the word "set" in a text, and he is unsure of its meaning within the context of the sentence. You show your friend how to look up the word using an online source, and you notice that it has a long list of meanings associated with it. Which of the following hints should you offer your friend to help him narrow down which definition might be the correct one?

   A. The correct meaning is usually the first definition listed in the entry.

   B. Use guide words to locate the word in a printed dictionary, which is likely more accurate.

   C. Determine how the word is functioning within the sentence, identify its part of speech, and find the definition(s) that match that part of speech.

   D. Find the connotative meaning of the word.

3. Look up the denotative meaning of the word "test," using an online or printed dictionary. Note the varied definitions, parts of speech, and word origins listed with this word. Compose a contextually correct sentence for at least two definitions of this word.

R.2.5 *Evaluate the author's purpose in a given text.*

This objective includes, but is not limited to, the following examples of knowledge, skills, and abilities.

- *Distinguish between fact and opinion.*
- *Summarize and compare information within a text.*
- *Recognize tone within context.*
- *Draw inferences about an author's purpose or message.*
- *Distinguish between informational, persuasive, expository, and entertaining.*

Key terms

anthology. A published collection of related works.

audience. The intended consumers of information.

authorial intent. The reason an author creates a text.

caption. Description of a figure or graphic.

publication. Printing or distribution of text.

Part of being an astute reader is determining the purpose of a piece of text. Determining an author's purpose, or the reason a particular piece of text was written, can help you focus on the most important details of a text. This is especially important if a text is very lengthy or complex. As you read, it is important to ask yourself whether the author is trying to persuade, inform, or entertain you. It is also important to remember that one text can have more than one purpose. In preparing for the TEAS, practice determining the author's purpose for all texts you encounter.

Knowing a writer's purpose (also called authorial intent) can be an important component of comprehension. If you want to understand a text deeply, it is helpful to know the circumstances under which it was produced.

When trying to determine authorial intent, it is helpful to ask yourself a series of questions as you read. Some especially helpful questions include the following.

Where does this text appear?

Is the text a novel, an excerpt from a novel, or a short story from an anthology? Does the text appear in a travel magazine plastered with images and advertisements for vendors associated with the area a writer is highlighting? Is the text a magazine or television advertisement? Where text appears can help you determine authorial intent.

If the text is in a newspaper, for example, the author might have intended to inform a community about issues pertinent to a specific geographical area. Novels, short stories, and poems are generally created to entertain an audience. Advertisements are created to persuade a group of people to make a purchase or act on a specific request.

Readers, however, must be careful to not assign a single purpose to any specific source. For example, while some news sources exist to inform readers, others were created to cater to a specific audience or set of beliefs. Likewise, many nonfiction texts that seek to inform readers can also be entertaining to read.

What is the structure of the text?

Structure can help you determine an author's intent. Below are some basic rules you can consider when examining the structure of a text.

Narrative

Narrative structures appear in stories or poetry, which often serve to entertain an audience. Narrative texts generally include a plot and one or more characters trying to overcome an obstacle or solve a problem.

Informational

While informational texts can take many forms, they often include section headings that might appear in bold or underlined type. Informational texts also often include bulleted or numbered lists, short phrases that might not be complete sentences, images with captions, maps, and diagrams. Instructions for assembly are an example of informational text. Course textbooks are another form of informational text. Both of these are used to inform readers about a specific topic.

Persuasive

Some persuasive texts are easy to recognize. Writers of advertisements seek to sell a service, product, or idea to a specific audience. Newspapers often include editorials that express specific opinions intended to persuade readers about a topic of local interest. However, some persuasive texts can be disguised. For example, Upton Sinclair wrote the novel *The Jungle*, which is widely read by many high school students today. But the fact that it is a work of fiction should not distract readers. Sinclair wrote it to inform a specific publication's audience about harsh working conditions inflicted upon American immigrants. *The Jungle* resulted in a public uproar about those poor working conditions and the lack of sanitation in the U.S. meat-packing industry in the early 1900s.

What is the author's tone?

Sometimes, an author's purpose can be determined by examining specific words used in a piece of writing. Authors who intend to simply inform readers tend to use straightforward, neutral language that lacks emotional correlation (words that can be defined as exclusively happy or exclusively angry). On the other hand, authors who intend to persuade readers might use emotionally-charged language coupled with images to evoke a specific emotion in readers. For example, an advertisement for a premium photo-printing service might ask potential customers, "How much are your memories worth?" These words, placed beneath an image of a grandparent smiling over a newborn child, might suggest that readers should not trust a local discount store to print their photos, but instead should use the advertiser's services. Paying attention to an author's words can help you determine the intended message.

R.2.5 Practice problems

Read the following excerpt from a small-town newspaper. Then, answer the question.

The rock star's appearance in town was brief but certainly noticeable. She visited a local child care center early Tuesday and then spent the afternoon visiting with area business owners and community leaders.

"It's refreshing to see that such a young lady who has achieved fame so early in life can still be a down-to-earth, compassionate, and caring person," said Chamber of Commerce President Karen Bitney.

The superstar wrapped up her visit by attending a Chamber dinner reception, at which she spoke about fostering youth leadership within a community. Following her speech, she announced a donation to a local food bank in the amount of $10,000.

1. What is the primary purpose of this text?
   A. To entertain readers with the story of the superstar's visit
   B. To entice readers to listen to the superstar's music
   C. To persuade readers to like the superstar
   D. To inform readers of the superstar's visit

2. Which of the following statements was written with a primary purpose to persuade readers?
   A. Fewer than 200 of these animals are in existence today. They have been nearing extinction since the early 1970s, and in the last 40 years their species has been even more threatened due to a decrease in their preferred habitat and an increase in predatory creatures.
   B. Fewer than 200 of these animals are in existence today. They have been nearing extinction since the early 1970s, and little attention from a handful of money-hungry legislators has resulted in few protections for these beloved animals. Your vote in November can help to ensure the preservation of thousands of dollars in funding that is guaranteed to protect these animals, as well as other endangered species around the world.
   C. Fewer than 200 of these animals are in existence today, so my camera crew was intent upon capturing every movement, every sound, and every nuanced emotion they could possibly glean through their lenses and microphones. We were in the African desert for 30 days, which sometimes seemed like a lifetime, but in retrospect was merely a blink.
   D. Fewer than 200 of these animals are in existence today, which makes them part of a long list of endangered species that our organization works every day to protect. While we would like to save every endangered species, our mission focuses primarily on species that number fewer than 250 worldwide.

3. Locate three texts that have different primary purposes: one each to inform, persuade, and entertain. Examine the qualities of each text, and determine the specific features that helped you to know which text was written for which purpose.

R.2.6 *Evaluate the author's point of view in a given text.*

This objective includes, but is not limited to, the following examples of knowledge, skills, and abilities.

- *Recognize different perspectives in text.*
- *Recognize and evaluate the text source (author, publication, organization).*
- *Compare texts from different sources and opinions.*
- *Evaluate the relevancy and accuracy of information.*
- *Gather, organize, and interpret information.*

Key terms

fact-checking. Verifying facts and statements in text.

peer-reviewed journal. Published writings that have been analyzed by experts in the field.

Developing the ability to determine an author's point of view can serve a reader well in the pursuit to gain a deep understanding of a text. Depending on the purpose of a text, an author's perspective (also known as an author's point of view) can be made very clear or it can remain intentionally hidden. For example, an editorial in a newspaper is intended to convey an author's perspective on a particular issue or topic. However, a news story written to inform a community about a serious recent tragedy is not supposed to include the writer's personal opinion about the event; the writer is simply meant to report the occurrence truthfully. For this TEAS task, you'll need to recognize and evaluate an author's point of view by thinking about who the author is, what organization(s) or group(s) he or she might be associated with, the type of publication in which a piece of writing appears, whether information the writer shares appears to be fact or opinion, and where a piece of writing "fits" within a larger context.

We might expect newspapers, news broadcasts, biographies, and documentaries to be sources of accurate and relevant information. Some of these sources take great pains to verify and fact-check information so that readers, viewers, and listeners can rely on them as sources of accurate information. However, all of these examples rely upon writers—human beings who by their very nature carry with them some biases and opinions that sometimes leak into their writing and reporting. It is important to some sources—various newspapers, for example—that a writer's opinion not interfere with the ability to report in a factual manner. However, some sources appear to be news sources but employ writers whose jobs are to share personal opinions, persuade readers about issues, and sometimes even deny readers' information that might sway them in a manner that goes against their purposes, beliefs, or sponsors' beliefs.

As you develop reading skills, it is important to identify the kinds of sources being read and discern the need for more information in order to develop a true and full understanding about a topic. For example, if reading a biography of George Washington in which a writer casts the first President as an arrogant, cruel, and harsh person, you might read another biography written by a different author. Although some of the information included in the book is bound to be the same, there will likely be additional information about another event in Washington's life, or a different take on an event covered in the first book you read that presents Washington as a kind and compassionate man rather than a cruel one. Seeing these differences in interpretations of a single man might cause you to look into who the authors are, their educational backgrounds, how they developed an interest in Washington, etc. Examining works by different authors about a single topic and comparing them can help you determine and better understand an author's point of view.

Sometimes researching background information about an author can help you to determine the point of view he or she might have, whether or not it is clear within a piece of writing. For example, in researching the benefits of using essential oils, you might stumble upon a blog that appears to be a source of useful, factual, and scientific information. However, when you click on the "About" tab at the top of the page and read about the blog's author, you discover that the author is the founder of a company that employs people to sell essential oils. Therefore, his ultimate purpose is likely to grow his business and entice the general public to use essential oils. This is not to say that the information included on his blog is untrue; much of it might very well be factual. However, you should be aware of the writer's probable purpose and seek out other sources of information in order to ensure that you have the most accurate information possible.

In the example, the fact that the writer was using a blog is also important to note. Blogs are widely used for a variety of purposes. Anyone can start a blog, and the information placed on one is generally not reviewed or verified to ensure accuracy. If you locate information on a blog, verify its accuracy by comparing it to other sources, especially those that have been reviewed by experts to ensure accuracy, such as peer-reviewed journals.

Relevance of information can also be an effective way to determine a writer's point of view. Political speeches illustrate this point nicely. In a political debate, for example, two candidates asked a variety of questions focused on diverse topics may consistently frame their answers around consistent themes. One candidate might mention the struggling middle class in each of her answers, while another candidate consistently mentions public safety in hers. While parts of their answers address the moderator's questions, they each consistently steer their answers back to topics they most want to discuss with voters. Analyzing the relevance or irrelevance of authors' (or speakers') information can be an effective way to determine his or her point of view.

R.2.6 Practice problems

1. You are reading reference letters for a candidate seeking employment with your business. Based on what you know about author's purpose, a reference letter from which of the following individuals is most likely to be accurate regarding the candidate's skills and ability to perform the job effectively?

   A. Candidate's previous employer

   B. Candidate's major advisor at his university

   C. Candidate's supervisor in a volunteer organization

   D. Candidate's longtime family friend

2. You are researching the effects of excessive consumption of diet carbonated beverages, specifically those containing artificial sweeteners such as aspartame. One online source you found indicates that there have been no proven side effects of large doses of aspartame in laboratory rats. Another online source argues that even small doses of aspartame in laboratory rats have caused neurological disorders and brain tumors. Where might you look within the sources to determine which author is presenting more reliable information?

   A. X-ray images of laboratory rats' brains located on the site indicating that aspartame causes brain tumors

   B. The "About" section, which lists information about each author's educational and professional background, as well as organizational affiliations

   C. Reviews from readers that are posted on each source's site

   D. Lists of links on each site that show where readers can go to obtain additional information

3. Do an online search for sites that cover a controversial topic that is of interest to you. Locate two sources that have differing opinions on the topic, and use your knowledge of author's perspective to determine which source is more reliable.

R.2.7 *Use text features.*

This objective includes, but is not limited to, the following examples of knowledge, skills, and abilities.

- *Find headings and subheadings.*
- *Identify features (e.g., key, legend, bold, italic, footnote, glossary, index, table of contents).*
- *Use navigational tools in media (e.g., search query, search engine).*

Text features are parts of a text that are designed to stand out from a larger text for a specific reason. Some examples of text features include bold print, italics, and footnotes. Text features can be used for a number of purposes, such as to orient the reader, provide additional information or background knowledge, assist a reader with quickly locating information, and provide a clear organizational structure. Good readers recognize text features and are able to use them effectively to better comprehend what they read. In order to do well with questions in this TEAS task, you should be able to locate headings and subheadings, identify various text features, and determine appropriate key words for searching a text or set of texts.

Headings and subheadings are some of the most common text features authors use to help readers understand how a text is organized.

In the example, "Summer 2015 Baseball and Softball" is the heading. "Eligibility" and "Game Locations and Times" are subheadings. Notice that the heading appears in bold type and is larger than the subheadings and the explanatory text. The subheadings also appear in bold type, but they are smaller. The subheadings and their explanations are indented to the right of the heading as well. Indentation is another text feature that helps to organize and clarify text for readers.

Summer 2015 Baseball and Softball

The city parks and recreation office is looking forward to a wonderful 2015 youth baseball and softball season. This year's sponsors are Bank of Sometown, AAA Office Supply Company, and Charlie's Dog Grooming.

Eligibility

Children entering grades 1-12 are eligible to play. All athletes must have a physical signed by a licensed physician on file with the office of parks and recreation at least one week prior to the start of the season.

Game Locations and Times

All games will be played at the city's recreation center, located at 543 Park Street. Games will be played Monday through Thursday, and a schedule with times will be posted to our parks and recreation website as soon as registrations are complete and team assignments are made.

Some text features are easily identified by where they appear on a page. Sidebars, footnotes, and map legends are some examples of these types of text features. Sidebars are often used in history textbooks. The main text in the book might focus on a world leader's work and major accomplishments associated with a particular social or political movement. A sidebar can include a photograph or image of the leader, along with an additional detail or two about her personal life.

Some other common text features are underlined and italicized print. These text features can be a bit more confusing to interpret because there are many reasons why text might be italicized or underlined. Likewise, formal style guides used by writers, reporters, and scholars use different sets of rules for italic and underlined print. It is sometimes up to a reader to infer why a portion of text appears different from the text around it. There are, however, some standard uses for text features. Italics, for example, are used for titles of works (e.g. books), foreign words or phrases, and for emphasis. A simple rule of thumb is that writers often use text features to draw attention to specific portions of text for specific reasons. Here are some simple questions you can ask yourself if you notice that part of a text has a different appearance than the text around it.

Sidebars like this one can offer readers additional information about a text that might not be provided in the main text.

- Is the text a title?
- Is the text a quotation that the author is using to help prove a point, introduce an idea, or make a statement?
- Is the text introducing a different section that will cover a new topic or idea?
- Is the text feature being used for aesthetic reasons only?
- Does the text feature help to organize information?
- Does the text feature have something to do with the type of text? (A script, for example, might include boldface type to indicate characters' names, and italics to indicate actions of characters.)

Footnotes are often used in informational texts to offer readers more in-depth information about a topic. Texts that use footnotes usually use numbers in superscript, or small numbers set slightly above the line of text. Here is an example:

> King Marshmallow held more wealth than any
> king in the land during his time.[4]

The example indicates that at the bottom of this page, readers can find additional information about this statement next to the number 4.

Map legends are a text feature invaluable to readers wanting to understand information included on a map. Legends often translate symbols included on a map in order to reduce clutter and make the map easier to read. For example, many maps indicate the population of towns and cities by assigning different styles of "dots" depending on the population range of a location. The legend, usually placed somewhere on the edge of the map, indicates which style of dot is assigned to each population range. Large urban centers with populations greater than 1 million people might be marked with a large black star with a circle around it, whereas very small towns might be marked with a tiny black dot. Rather than be left to guess about what each symbol means, readers can look to the legend for help with interpretation.

Effectively interpreting text features will help you to read a text more accurately and efficiently. Additionally, knowing what kinds of text features might appear in a text can also help you locate information. For example, if you are searching for a scholarly article about the spread of contagious disease among school children, you might think about what subheadings would exist within articles, and use those words as search terms in your research.

Text features help add meaning to texts that readers might not otherwise understand. Bold type, italics, indention, underlining, sidebars, legends, and footnotes are some common text features that readers might encounter. Paying attention to why texts appear the way they do can help you gain additional knowledge when reading.

Key terms

aesthetic. Guiding principles of a piece of work.

footnote. Comment at the bottom of a page that refers to something within the text.

heading. A title.

query. A question.

search engine. Website to locate information online.

search term. Words used to find information via a search engine.

style guide. Set of conventions and standards for a type of writing.

subheading. A title of a subdivision of information with a larger text.

superscript. Text that is smaller and above the surrounding text.

R.2.7 Practice problems

1. Which of the following identifies why the following passage includes italicized print?

   In his most recent work, *Free Popcorn Under the Bleachers!*, Mr. Andrews offers readers a humorous account of his childhood, growing up as the youngest of eight children.

   A. It is an advertisement.

   B. It is a subheading.

   C. It is a footnote.

   D. It is a book title.

2. A team you work with is hosting a fundraiser for a local hospital and needs help with promotional flyers advertising the event. The information they have included seems disorganized and unclear. Which of the following text features could help to organize the flyer in its current form?

   We need your help!

   Saturday, July 18th
   8:00 a.m.

   $50 per person

   Bring your pets!

   See map below.

   Fundraiser for local hospital

   Anytown Memorial Hospital, north parking lot

   Breakfast and Fun Run

   All proceeds will be donated to AMH.

   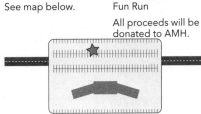

   A. Italicized print, sidebar, colored text, and footnotes

   B. Bold type, indentation, headings, subheadings, and legend

   C. Legend, footnotes, and italicized print

   D. Sidebar and legend

3. Locate three texts, and identify and evaluate the text features within them. Then answer the following questions pertaining to the text features you locate.

   A. What are the text features included in this text?

   B. What is the purpose of each of the text features the authors of these texts use?

   C. What additional text features might be appropriate for these texts that could lead to deeper or richer understanding for readers?

Practice problem answers

R.2.1

1. Option C is correct because the statement can be proven true or false. Options B and D are biases because they are preferential viewpoints with little allowance for discussion. Option A might be a proven aspect of obesity, but is not the only proven cause of obesity. The emotionally-charged use of inappropriate also connotes opinion.

2. Even though there is a positive connotation with the word incredible, this is still a stereotype that makes a generalization about Japanese individuals. This is harmful because it makes an assumption that will not always be correct and omits individuality and diversity.

3. Option B is correct because the author uses words such as hardships, tragedies, and follies to demonstrate a negative picture. In addition, the author explicitly states that "we should shake our heads at their foolishness, and transfer our admiration to people who have made real discoveries." While the author does use the word "memorable" to describe Franklin's expedition, he also categorizes it as a "disaster." The author's critique of arctic explorations does not accord with the idea that adventure is an adequate reason to risk the hardships of arctic exploration. While the author does indicate that arctic exploration should be abandoned until a safer means is available, the absolute "never" does not best align with the author's point of view.

R.2.2

1. Option B is correct. This is evident through the introductory statement "All that to the side" and the quote "I think you should consider." Option A is incorrect because although the author shows some points about Alex's strength, his purpose is to persuade Debra to hire him. Option C is incorrect because there is no descriptive language or a narrative order of sequence. Option D is incorrect because descriptive is a type, not a mode.

2. Option C is correct because it signals a comparison of differences. Options A and D show similarities. Option B signals a cause-and-effect relationship, but this passage is about differences.

3. The reason answers why to a claim. It gives the reader more clarification as to why the reader should agree or understand the claim. The evidence shows what the claim looks like. In other words, it supports the claim with facts or details.

R.2.3

1. Option C is correct because the combined use of terrible grating sound, absolute finality, and apprehensive connote a collective mood of nervousness. Options B and D are incorrect because the connotation of nervousness overpowers the feelings of excitement and fear. The shipmates overcame their fear to follow their captain. Option A is incorrect because the setting might be adventurous, but the narrator's tone was one of nervousness as illustrated by word choice.

2. Option A is correct because foolishness connotes a negative feeling of injudiciousness and imprudence. The other words all have positive connotations.

3. Option D is correct because this is a prime example of a word's definition mentioned in the same passage. The other options are synonyms that lack specific contextual meaning.

R.2.4

1. Option B is correct. "apt" comes after "app" and before "avi" alphabetically.
   - "apt" comes after both "ane" and "ant" alphabetically.
   - "apt" comes after both "all" and "apo" alphabetically.
   - "apt" comes before both "are" and "arm" alphabetically.

2. Option C is correct. Knowing the part of speech, or how the word is functioning within the sentence, should help narrow down the list.
   - The sentence in which this word appears might not feature the most common use of the word.
   - It is likely that the paper dictionary would include identical definitions to the online source.
   - Determining the connotative meaning—or additional, implied meaning—for this word will not help.

R.2.5

1. Option D is correct. The author presents information in a factual, even tone and comments on the superstar's whereabouts without including personal opinions about her actions.
   - This passage lacks the tone and narrative that one would expect if the primary purpose was to entertain.
   - The passage does not include any information or judgment about the superstar's music.
   - While the passage contains information about the superstar that some readers might find to be positive, the information is of a factual nature. The author does not use language that indicates any feelings about the superstar.

2. Option B is correct. This option cites statistics, includes emotionally charged language ("money-hungry legislators"), and contains a direct request for readers to vote a particular way in an upcoming election.
   - Option A cites statistics about the animals and their predators, but contains no emotionally charged language or statement about how the author personally feels about their looming extinction.
   - Option C is a first-person narrative account of an author's experience with these animals. The writer is not seeking to persuade a reader, but rather to tell a story.
   - Option D is a statement about an organization's purpose and mission. While one might assume that such an organization would happily accept donations or seek support for their cause, this particular excerpt is merely informing readers about the organization's purpose.

R.2.6

1. Option A is correct. This person is likely to know the most about the candidate's work habits, work quality, and abilities to perform well on the job.
   - Option B has a vested interest in his students gaining employment, so it is likely that a reference letter from this source will be biased in favor of the candidate.
   - While it is likely a good sign that this candidate volunteers his time to benefit others, option C benefits from the candidate's commitment, so it is unlikely that the supervisor will offer an entirely unbiased account of the candidate's work.
   - It is not likely that option D knows much about the work habits or work quality of the candidate. While the friend might feel she is being truthful about the candidate, she is likely to be biased in favor of the candidate because she cares about him personally.
2. Option B is correct. This will tell you whether the author is qualified to be making the claims he is making. The organizational affiliations will help you to know if the information presented might be biased in a way to not compromise profits or membership for a particular organization.
   - While option A might be interesting information, it will not prove that this author is more or less reliable than the other.
   - Ordinarily, owners/writers of websites have the ultimate say in what is displayed on their site. While some readers might truthfully say wonderful things about the author and the source, it is not clear whether the author is editing reviews or perhaps not posting reviews he does not find favorable.
   - While a list of links will be helpful if you choose to do more research, the links are likely to be those that agree with each source's perspective.

R.2.7

1. Option D is correct. It is set off as an appositive to "his most recent work" and is the title of Mr. Andrews' book.
   - This portion of italicized print appears as part of a larger sentence. Its context indicates that it is not an advertisement.
   - The italicized print does not serve to organize the text in any way, as subheadings do.
   - Footnotes are included at the bottom of a page of text, separate from a main text. This portion of italicized print appears as part of a larger sentence.
2. Option B is correct. This flyer needs a good deal of help, and these four text features will likely do the trick. Organizing the words with headings and subheadings that appear in bold type and are indented to help readers interpret which information helps them know where to go vs. which information is about the fundraiser's cause will be helpful. Also, including a legend for the map will help readers understand what the red triangle, yellow stars, and blue boxes show.
   - Italicized print, a sidebar, and colored text might create a more attractive and informational flyer, but those text features alone will likely not be sufficient for making the flyer clear to readers. Footnotes do not seem appropriate for this text.
   - While a legend and some italicized print might be a step in the right direction, footnotes do not seem appropriate here. Overall, these three text features will likely not be enough to make the flyer entirely clear for readers.
   - A legend for the map seems appropriate, and perhaps a sidebar could offer potential donors some additional information, but these two text features alone will likely not be enough to make the flyer entirely clear for readers.

R.3.1 *Identify primary sources in various media.*

Primary sources exist in all types of media. The term "primary source documents" refers to artifacts, letters, recordings, images, and other media that have not been altered from their original state. They are created by individuals within a specific context. This task requires you to know the meaning of "primary source document," distinguish between primary source and other types of documents, and be able to locate information within primary source documents.

When trying to determine whether something is a primary source, it can be helpful to think of sources in terms of how close they are to the creator. This is sometimes referred to as "degrees of separation." If the source itself is the only thing separating the reader from its creator, then the source is considered a primary source document. It is also helpful to understand that the same source could be considered a primary source OR part of a secondary or tertiary source, depending on how you access it.

For example, original photographs taken by an embedded war photojournalist are primary source documents, provided that you are viewing actual prints. These actual prints would most likely be found in a museum or library. However, if these photographs were purchased by a textbook company and included in a chapter to help students gain a better understanding of a military conflict, they would no longer be considered primary source documents.

To further complicate matters, many primary source documents include secondary sources within them. The U.S. Declaration of Independence is a wonderful example of this. The authors included information within that document about the wrongs imposed upon them by the British government. This information would be considered secondary sources, and possibly even tertiary sources.

Although it can seem complicated to determine whether some sources can be called primary source documents, some sources are almost always considered primary. Artifacts, such as ancient tools or ancient artwork, are almost always considered primary sources. If we ask ourselves, "How many degrees of separation are there between the creator of this and me?" it is easy to see why ancient artwork, archaeological artifacts, and things of that nature are usually considered primary sources. It is likely that the only thing standing between you and the creator is the artifact itself. So with one degree of separation, it is clearly a primary source. Usually, primary source documents are used to gain valuable information about a specific time or place.

This objective includes, but is not limited to, the following examples of knowledge, skills, and abilities.

- *Identify primary sources.*

- *Recognize primary source materials (e.g., Internet, video, text, audio, artifact, print media, photograph, autobiography, document, memoir, oral history).*

- *Locate information in a primary source.*

Key terms

degrees of separation. Number of steps removed from an origin.

primary source. A firsthand document or source created at the time in question.

secondary source. Secondhand account of events.

tertiary source. A compilation of primary and secondary sources.

R.3.1 Practice problems

1. Which of the following is a primary source document?

   A. A textbook containing original photographs purchased directly from photojournalists

   B. Diaries of WWII prisoners of war

   C. Diary entries of WWII prisoners of war printed in a newspaper in honor of Veterans Day

   D. A newspaper article retelling one town's history with violent acts

2. Which of the following is generally true regarding primary source documents?

   A. Ancient artifacts such as handmade weapons and tools are almost always considered primary sources.

   B. A document is either wholly a primary source document or not.

   C. Textbooks almost always use primary source documents.

   D. Primary sources only refer to print documents.

3. Visit a library near you and ask a library media specialist to help you locate some primary source documents. What do the sources you find teach you about the people who created them? What might be lost if this primary source were to be described or photographed for use within another source?

R.3.2 *Use evidence from text to make predictions and inferences, and draw conclusions about a piece of writing.*

This objective includes, but is not limited to, the following examples of knowledge, skills, and abilities.

- *Synthesize information from the text to form a prediction, make an inference, and form a conclusion.*

- *Cite evidence from the text to support a prediction, inference, or conclusion.*

Key terms

foreshadowing. An author's hints of events to come.

prediction. A reader's guess of events to come.

Often, writers leave out certain details about a story or topic, and it is up to readers to put together details from a text to draw conclusions about the author's intended meaning. Readers draw conclusions by making reasonable inferences and predictions based on details they find in a text. Being able to cite specific evidence explaining how you came to a conclusion will help you to gain credibility as a reader, and can be a benefit to others wanting to better understand a writer's work. For this TEAS task, you will need to be able to successfully identify evidence from a text to support predictions, inferences, and conclusions.

Fiction writers sometimes provide vague details about a character or situation as a narrative strategy, or to build a sense of mystery within a text. In these instances, writers expect readers to ask questions, form hypotheses, and draw on potentially important details to predict characters' actions, plot twists, and story resolutions. One literary technique fiction authors use to help readers predict is foreshadowing.

Suppose an author begins a story with the line, "If I had known I would end up in the hospital, I never would have called him back." This opening line alone captures readers' attention and creates a situation in which readers are inferring and predicting what might have happened to the narrator. Did she have a bad date? Did she call back someone who lured her into harm's way? Readers can make reasonable predictions about what might have happened based on details introduced in this opening line.

"The young spectacled boy stood in the corner, looking down at the gym floor, shuffling his feet. He had told his mother to pick him up when the dance ended at 9:30, but he was already regretting that decision; it was only 7:45. Little did he know that 8:00 would bring an event that would not only change his fate for the evening, but change the course of his life forever."

An inference is like a prediction, but can be more subtle. While readers of this passage might predict that something significant will happen to this young boy within the next 15 minutes, readers might also infer some details about the boy's personality. "Stood in the corner, looking down ... shuffling his feet" indicates that he feels shy or nervous in this social situation. He is also alone, indicating that his friends did not come to the dance, or he has no friends.

Good readers also make predictions, inferences, and conclusions about informational pieces of writing. Sometimes, the structure of a text can assist readers in making predictions about what an author will include. If the text includes a numbered list, a reader might predict that the author will be giving instructions in a sequence, or providing a list of items in order of their importance. A title is a text feature that can also help readers make predictions about what might be included.

One thing readers often must infer in all types of texts is word meanings. When readers stumble across an unknown word, they might make an educated guess about its meaning before consulting a dictionary. Often, words that surround an unknown word can provide readers clues about the meaning of a word.

Whether or not writers intend their readers to predict, infer, and draw conclusions, it is likely that every text at some point will require a reader to do these things. In a sense, all readers are experimenters, trying out words, exploring meanings, and predicting events and outcomes.

R.3.2 Practice problems

The grandmothers met every year. It was tradition. They'd been meeting every year since they'd left home at the age of 12 to work, attend school, and eventually marry and start families of their own. Their father had hoped they would remain close, even though he was forced to send them away; their mother had cried out of fear that they would never know one another well, and out of fear that their families might exist as complete strangers in the world.

But the grandmothers knew better. Even at age 12, they both had a feeling that even though they had to be separated for a while, they would eventually come back to one another and be closer than ever before. How did they know this? Some say it was magic. Some believe it was a sixth sense that sisters seem to have about such things. But they will tell you to this day that it was one thing and one thing only: the shed.

1. Which of the following might indicate that the sisters were forced apart by poverty?

   A. Their father "was forced to send them away."

   B. "They would eventually come back to one another and be closer than ever before."

   C. "The grandmothers met every year."

   D. "Their mother had cried…"

2. Which of the following is a reasonable conclusion about what the author will include in the pages to follow?

   A. Information about their father's profession and what caused them to be poor

   B. Accounts of sisters in other families who seem to have a sixth sense about one another

   C. Information about their mother, who suffered from depression

   D. Information about the significance and history of the shed, and a moment the grandmothers shared there when they were young, prior to leaving their family home

3. Read the first page of any work of fiction. Infer some details about the character(s), setting, or conflict. Make a prediction about what will be included in subsequent pages.

R.3.3 *Compare and contrast themes from print and other sources.*

This objective includes, but is not limited to, the following examples of knowledge, skills, and abilities.

- *List similarities and differences across themes.*
- *Recognize similar themes across cultures.*
- *Compare and contrast a theme from one author or topic.*
- *Compare and contrast themes across genres.*

Key terms

genre. A group of related writings or other media.

social commentary. Use of rhetoric to make statements about current culture.

social structure. The system and relationships between groups of society.

theme. A foundational concept engaged with by a piece of art.

A theme is a broad concept, often thought of as a universal concern, that an author addresses through a given medium. This is distinct from the specific subject matter of, for example, a piece of writing. While the subject matter of a story might be a specific crime, the primary theme of the work could be social inequality. How that theme plays out in the specific context of the story will inform our understanding of the crime and the larger story. This task requires several skills: finding similarities and differences between themes, recognizing similar themes across different cultures, comparing and contrasting the way in which a single author uses a theme, comparing and contrasting different themes related to a topic, and comparing and contrasting how a theme appears across different genres.

Themes are present in both short and long works of fiction and nonfiction, as well as with nonprint sources such as films and radio broadcasts. Sometimes themes are obvious because a work has a specific purpose or aim, such as to convince a person or group of people about a point of view on a topic. However, themes can be less obvious and require a reader to pull together different parts of a text in order to recognize them. When reading a story, watching a film, or looking at an artwork, ask yourself: What are the big ideas that the artist is engaging with? How are those concepts addressed?

Novels can engage with a number of themes and do so in a number of ways. This explains why two teachers can teach books in completely different ways. One teacher of Harper Lee's *To Kill a Mockingbird* might choose to highlight the injustices experienced by the African-American community in the 1930s, while another teacher might focus on the presence of social hierarchies during that time period.

Some common themes across classic works of literature often studied in the U.S. are power, motherhood, freedom, and privilege. Much can be learned from the themes present within the works of literature in a particular culture, geographic area, or even time period. Recurring themes of oppression within the literature of a time period or culture would likely indicate an oppressive regime or social structure. Presence of a single theme across genres and authors can often signal a historically significant event or attitude among a group of people.

While a theme can sometimes be treated in a similar manner by different authors, authors often take different perspectives on a single theme. For example, the theme of motherhood is present in many works of fiction and nonfiction, but different authors have different messages for their readers about motherhood. It is important to recognize that authors can treat the same theme very differently within works of fiction or nonfiction. Often, genre will impact how a theme is addressed. A romantic comedy, for instance, will take a much more light-hearted approach to the theme of love than a tragedy like *Romeo and Juliet*.

Films are a wonderful medium in which to note powerful themes, and filmmakers choose to display and comment on themes in many ways. For example, a director might choose to highlight the powerlessness of a certain group of people by using camera angles that look down on a group of people rather than a head-on or from below. Camera angles showing a subject from below can depict a character as more powerful or important than those around her. Scenes that show a subject as a very small part of the screen in comparison with a vast landscape can also depict a theme of powerlessness.

Once you become adept at finding themes in all artistic genres, you will more easily be able to evaluate one author or artist's treatment of a theme in relation to another. Likewise, you can begin to look at themes as social commentary and analyze them in relation to cultural or historic movements that might have influenced an artist.

R.3.3 Practice problems

1. Which of the following are ways in which both print and nonprint sources express themes?

   A. Repetition and prominence

   B. Camera angles

   C. Lighting

   D. Length of the work

2. Which of the following is true about themes?

   A. They typically occur only once within a print source.

   B. They only exist in print media.

   C. They can reveal information about a specific culture or time period.

   D. Different artists' or authors' treatments of a single theme should not be compared.

3. Locate a newspaper article, fiction short story, and piece of artwork (painting, drawing, cartoon, sculpture) from similar time periods. Are there any themes in common among the three pieces you selected? If so, what are they and why might that theme be present in more than one piece? Is there historical significance to the theme you have found?

R.3.4 *Evaluate an argument and its specific claims.*

Key terms

argument. A set of reasons to make a case for an idea.

claim. A statement that something is true.

research-based. Reliant upon ideas backed by study.

support. Lend credibility to an idea.

valid. Proven as true.

The word "argument" can certainly be a synonym for the word "conflict," but in writing it often means something a bit different. An author's argument is essentially a point that an author believes or seems to believe is true. The argument is what is stated, and the author often will provide reasons—or evidence—that support the argument. In order to do well with this TEAS task, you will need to be able to identify an author's argument and supporting evidence, and examine the information that supports the argument to determine its relevance and sufficiency.

Locating a writer's argument, sometimes called a claim, is usually not difficult. When you are reading a text and being asked to do or believe something, that "something" is the author's argument. Sometimes an author's argument is preceded by words like "I think" or "I believe." However, strong argumentative pieces usually do not include those clue words; instead, an author creates a solid argument by simply stating that something is or should be true.

It is not enough, however, for a writer to simply state an argument or make a claim. He should also have evidence to support why the argument is true or valid. Reasons are often stated following an argument, but some authors might purposely place their main argument at the end of a piece after they have stated all the reasons readers should agree with their perspective. Evidence can be directly or indirectly related to the claim, but it will definitely provide readers reasons to agree with the author.

Some evidence is better than others. Evidence drawn from sources that are known to be reputable and based on sound research will likely be more reliable and help to support an argument better than evidence drawn from sources that are not. When evaluating sources, ask yourself who the author(s) are, whether the source is peer reviewed, how new the source is, and whether that makes a difference to the argument it is being used to support.

Some authors also use evidence that is somewhat unrelated to the argument. While this might be accidental, sometimes presenting unrelated evidence is a strategy. When you are evaluating the validity of an argument and its evidence, think about how closely the evidence aligns with the argument being presented. If the evidence is inconsequential or out of alignment with the argument, perhaps the author does not have enough support for his position.

Recognizing an author's argument and corresponding evidence is important. Readers who can distinguish between strong and weak arguments and evidence will be ultimately better informed about issues important to them.

R.3.4 Practice problems

Dear Fellow Community Residents,

It has recently come to my attention that a local restaurant—one that has been a favorite of my own friends and family for generations—needs our help.

Bob's Brownie Barn, a staple of many families' dessert tables since our great-grandparents first arrived in town, has recently been cited for mold infestation in several places throughout the restaurant. The health department has forced the owners to close their doors until a subsequent inspection reveals that all harmful toxins have been removed from the premises. A recent bid revealed that complete eradication of the mold will cost between $10,000 and $15,000, an amount utterly unmanageable for the owners.

We need to rally behind this community icon and work together to save the Brownie Barn. Although $10,000 might seem like a large sum, in our community of 12,000, if each of us gave just $1, the owners would likely have more than enough to pay for the cleanup. Though the cleanup is their responsibility, it is believed that this mold infestation is result of the previous upstairs tenant's unkempt living quarters, which the Brownie Barn neither owns nor controls. The Brownie Barn has been a frequent donor for events in and around this community for the past 60 years, and now it is our turn to step up and assist this important community business.

Those wishing to donate can call or stop by Community Bank and request to deposit to the Bob's Brownie Barn mold account. It will be open for deposits until all necessary funds are raised. Please keep in mind the urgency of this situation, however. The owners operate this business as a primary source of income and have been closed for more than 2 weeks now. The time to donate is now.

Sincerely,

Pete Saenz, Brownie Lover

1. What is the writer's main argument?

   A. Bob's Brownie Barn is important to the community.

   B. Community members should donate money to help the owners of Bob's Brownie Barn.

   C. The community has loved Bob's Brownie Barn for at least three generations.

   D. $10,000 is not very much money.

2. Which of the following is evidence the writer provides to support his main argument?

   A. The tenants above the Brownie Barn have moved out.

   B. Most of the families living in the community today have lived in the community for several generations.

   C. The Community Bank is an example of good will.

   D. The Brownie Barn has been a frequent donor to various community causes.

3. Find and view a political speech delivered by a candidate, or download a transcription of a political speech of a candidate seeking office. Consider the speaker's main argument to be "vote for me," and locate within the speech all the evidence intended to support this primary argument.

R.3.5 *Evaluate and integrate data from multiple sources in various formats, including media.*

This objective includes, but is not limited to, the following examples of knowledge, skills, and abilities.

- *Synthesize data from texts, charts, or graphs.*
- *Organize data from various sources.*
- *Examine various data sources.*
- *Combine data from various sources into one document.*
- *Select relevant data.*

Key terms

chart. A type of diagram that graphically represents data.

diagram. A symbolic representation of information.

graph. A type of diagram that mathematically displays data.

information specialist. A library employee who helps patrons find information.

library media specialist. A library employee who helps patrons find media sources.

professional journal. Published periodical texts that represent a specific industry.

People read information about topics that interest them on a regular basis, often in newspapers, magazines, professional journals, blogs, and—of course—books. Sometimes these sources include charts, graphs, and diagrams that help to explain an idea shared in a text. If multiple sources of information are not already included in a particular text, it is often a good idea to locate additional sources that could provide more information about a topic. Doing so will ensure that you develop a more complete understanding of an issue, which will leave you better equipped to converse with others or write more meaningfully on the topic. Most documents produced in postsecondary coursework and by professionals require the author to integrate knowledge from multiple sources. This TEAS task will test your ability to synthesize, organize, and analyze data from multiple sources.

Whatever the topic, it is usually wise to seek multiple data sources so that an understanding can be based on multiple perspectives. For example, imagine you are a health professional and a client has come to you seeking clearance to participate in a study of a new medication to regulate blood pressure. You might begin with an initial question: **What data is most relevant to you?** You would probably want a history of the patient's blood pressure, plus any other related health information. You would likely examine the patient yourself in her current state and gather data about her height, weight, heart rate, medications, and other basic health information.

This initial question and round of data-gathering will likely lead you to ask another question: **What additional sources of information could help you?** You might know some additional sources of information already, depending on how knowledgeable you are about the topic. However, if you have trouble thinking of additional information sources, library media specialists can be excellent resources. Sometimes also known as information specialists, they can assist with finding information relevant to a wealth of questions and topics. For the purposes of our example, you might be interested in finding information about negative impacts of traditional blood pressure medications on clients who have various health afflictions, some of which your client might have.

Once you have determined the information you need and located several sources to provide that information, the next step is to organize the information in a logical manner. One way to do this is by using a coding system that makes sense to you. For the purposes of our example, you might mark articles or patient data related to body mass index with the letters BMI, and articles and patient data related to heart rate with HR. Marking information can help physically sort it into physical or electronic folders so you can come back to it when you need it.

There are many technology tools that can help organize information in meaningful ways. These tools can help people organize articles, data, and notes into electronic files and folders. Using technology to help organize information can save money by eliminating printing costs and time sorting through pages of information in order to locate what is most relevant.

After organizing the information, ask yourself, **How does all of this fit together and what does it mean?** This stage is often called "synthesis" because you have taken information from many sources, pulled it apart and thought about it, and now you must put it all back together in a meaningful way. For the purposes of our example, your recommendation will be supported by data you have gathered about the patient and outside sources that provide guidance on best practices related to this particular instance.

Gathering, organizing, analyzing, evaluating, and synthesizing information from multiple sources is an invaluable skill in many professions. Developing the ability to use multiple sources to make decisions and respond to situations helps to ensure more sound and thoughtful actions.

R.3.5 Practice problems

You are a member of the Human Resources staff at ABC Company, and have been asked to look into why Mr. Jim Grotten, a longtime employee of the company, has declining numbers of new clients. In order to assist in your investigation, your supervisor has provided you four pieces of information, including a graph showing Grotten's absences over the past 3 months, a graph showing the number of new clients Grotten has signed in the past 3 months, results from client satisfaction surveys for Grotten's existing clients over the past 3 months, and a recent email from one of Grotten's existing clients.

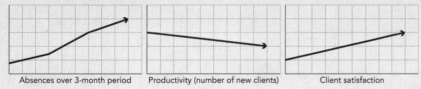

Absences over 3-month period   Productivity (number of new clients)   Client satisfaction

Subject: Jim G.

From: Carla Cox, CEO of XYZ Company

To: Benjamin Best, CEO of ABC Company

Hello, Mr. Best. I wanted to send you a quick note of appreciation in regard to a recent meeting I had with Jim Grotten, my sales representative with ABC Company. I've been working with Jim for almost 10 years now, and can say with confidence that he is the sole reason I do not explore other options for servicing XYZ Company. He is competent, attentive, and knows what services will suit the needs of my customers. I've had outstanding offers from other vendors that would save my company money in the short term. However, I don't want to imagine what would happen to us if we did not have Jim in our corner.

Thank you for continuing to offer a quality service for my company, and thank you for doing what it takes to retain employees like Jim. We look forward to many more years of working with him and with ABC Company.

Sincerely,

Carla Cox, CEO of XYZ Company

1. Which of the following information sources present a potentially negative picture of Mr. Grotten?

   A. Data on employee absences and data on productivity

   B. Data on productivity and data from client satisfaction survey

   C. Data from client satisfaction survey and email from current client

   D. Email from current client and data on employee absences

2. Which of the following data seems to rely entirely on Mr. Grotten to improve?

   A. Employee absences

   B. Productivity

   C. Client satisfaction survey results

   D. Complimentary emails from clients

3. Imagine you are asked to make a decision about whether to fire Mr. Grotten. What additional information would you need in order to feel comfortable with your choice?

Practice problem answers

R.3.1

1. Option B is correct. These are primary source documents because the diaries are the only thing separating the reader from the writer.
   - Because readers will access the photos from a textbook rather than look at the photos separate from the textbook source, these photographs are not primary source documents.
   - Because readers would access these diary entries in a format divorced from the state in which they were created, they are not primary source documents.
   - If there were artifacts or documents written by those who lived through the violent acts, those artifacts or documents would be primary sources. An article written about them and the time period in which they existed is not a primary source document.
2. Option A is correct. These artifacts provide a direct link between people today and those in the past who created the artifacts.
   - Some sources can be both primary or secondary, depending on how readers or viewers access them.
   - Option B might be true for some textbook vendors, but this is not a rule or a known fact.
   - Primary sources can exist in all different media, including print and nonprint.

R.3.2

1. Option A is correct. This is the strongest piece of evidence to suggest that the family was too poor to care for two young girls.
   - Option B does not suggest anything about their financial state prior to or at the time of leaving.
   - Option C does not suggest anything about their financial state prior to or at the time of leaving.
   - While option D indicates that their mother was upset, the text suggests that she was upset that the girls might never really know one another, not that they were poor.
2. Option D is correct. The passage foreshadows that this shed holds significance for the grandmothers and that the reason why will be included in subsequent pages.
   - The text indicates that the main information to come will be about how the grandmothers came to know they would meet every year, and it has something to do with a shed.
   - The text includes option B as a detail, but makes no indication that this will be a primary focus in the pages to come.
   - Although the text states their mother was upset when the girls went away, there is no indication that the pages to come will be primarily about their mother. There is also no evidence that the mother suffered from depression.

R.3.3

1. Option A is correct. Both writers and artists express themes by repeating ideas or images, or by giving one idea or image prominence within a work.
   - Option B can be true for videographers, but writers do not use cameras, so this would not work for print sources.
   - Option C can be true for visual artists, but writers would have to describe light rather than use it.
   - Themes can appear in both long and short works, but the length typically does not have any bearing on what themes are present. This also would not pertain as readily to stationary visual art, such as paintings and drawings.
2. Option C is correct. Common themes that reoccur throughout literature and artwork of a particular culture or time period can reveal information about beliefs, attitudes, and afflictions of people within that culture or time period.
   - In order for a theme to be recognized, it must be prominent within a source, which typically means that it is repeated multiple times throughout the work.
   - Though themes exist differently in non-print media, they are definitely present.
   - Readers and viewers can learn a great deal by comparing and contrasting how different artists and authors develop the same theme within their work.

R.3.4

1. Option B is correct. This is the primary argument and the main purpose of this letter.
   - Options A and C are pieces of evidence the writer provides, but neither is his main argument.
   - Option D is a tactic the writer uses to convince readers of his main argument, but it is not his main argument.
2. Option D is correct. The author offers this as evidence that community members should repay the favor and donate to help the Brownie Barn, just as its owners have helped the community in the past.
   - Though option A seems to be true and seems indirectly related to the argument, it is an aside and is not mentioned as evidence to support the main argument that community members should donate money to the Brownie Barn.
   - Though option B is suggested in the letter, it is not directly connected to the main argument and therefore is not evidence to support the main argument.
   - One might conclude option C is true based on the fact that the bank is hosting an account for donors to deposit funds into, but this statement is not offered as support for the main argument.

R.3.5

1. Option A is correct. The graph of absences shows that Mr. Grotten's absences have increased over the past 3 months. Likewise, the productivity graph shows that the number of new clients Mr. Grotten has signed has decreased over the past 3 months.
   - While the data on productivity could be viewed negatively, the satisfaction of clients appears to have increased over the past 3 months, according to the graph.
   - Both of the pieces of information in option C reflect favorably on Mr. Grotten.
   - The email from the current client reflects favorably on Mr. Grotten, but the graph showing an increase in his absences might reflect poorly on him.
2. Option A is correct. Decreasing the number of absences seems within the control of Mr. Grotten.
   - Outside factors, such as new clients' budgets, could play a role in whether they sign on as new clients.
   - Some clients might not complete the survey, or some might have a biased impression of Mr. Grotten.
   - Mr. Grotten has no control over whether his clients send emails about him.

Reading section quiz

The next six questions are based on this passage.

Call Options Explained

Most investors are comfortable buying and selling stocks, but only a few understand stock options. Options are more complex than stocks, and many books have been written on the topic. However, a few options basics can be explained in the space of several paragraphs.

A call option is a contract that allows a person to buy a stock at a fixed price, within a fixed time frame.

Example: Stock XYZ is currently trading at $50. Sharon believes that stock XYZ will go up sometime in the next month. She therefore buys call options that entitle her to buy 500 shares of XYZ at a price of $50 sometime in the next month. She pays a small amount of money, called the premium, to get those options.

A month later, Sharon will take action based on what stock XYZ has done.

Case A: Stock XYZ has indeed climbed; it now trades at $70 a share. Sharon therefore exercises her right to buy 500 shares of XYZ at $50. Because the current market price of XYZ is $70, Sharon can then immediately sell her shares on the open market, earning $20 of profit per share.

Case B: Stock XYZ didn't climb; instead, it fell to $30 a share. In this case, Sharon's options have become worthless, because nobody wants to pay $50 for shares that are currently worth only $30. She therefore does nothing, letting her options expire.

Why did Sharon bother buying options at all, instead of simply buying shares of stock XYZ? The answer lies in Case B: the price of XYZ plummeted, but instead of losing a great deal of money, Sharon only lost the small premium she paid for her options. Call options allowed her to bet on the market without taking on too much risk.

1. Which of the following examples is a concise summary of the passage?
   A. Call options are an immediate way to make money when investing.
   B. Call options allow for low-risk stock market investment.
   C. Making call options is more complex than typical investing.
   D. In order to be a successful investor, one must purchase call options.

2. Which of the following is a logical conclusion of the passage?
   A. A call option allows an investor to purchase a stock at a fixed price, within a fixed time frame.
   B. Sometimes stocks climb and sometimes they fall.
   C. Investors should understand what call options are and be aware of the low-risk opportunities call options offer.
   D. Sharon made a good choice in buying the options.

3. Which of the following defines a call option?
   A. A call option can be explained in the space of several paragraphs.
   B. A call option is Sharon's best option for purchase.
   C. A call option is a contract that allows a person to buy a stock at a fixed price within a fixed time frame.
   D. A call option is when Sharon pays a premium.

4. Which of the following sentences correctly describes Sharon's sequence of events?
   A. Sharon's option is worthless and she does nothing.
   B. Sharon exercises her right to buy 500 shares of XYZ at $50; then she immediately sells her shares on the open market.
   C. First she pays a premium, then buys her call options, and finally takes action.
   D. She buys call options then takes action later.

5. Which of the following best describes the mode of this passage?
   A. Expository
   B. Descriptive
   C. Persuasive
   D. Narrative

6. Which of the following is the purpose of this selection?
   A. Entertain
   B. Inform
   C. Persuade
   D. Describe

Mom's Scalloped Potato Dish

Ingredients

½ pound thinly sliced potatoes

2-3 onions, roughly chopped

1 can evaporated milk

3 cups grated cheese

Steps

Preheat oven to 350 degrees.

Mix potatoes and onions.

Put ⅔ of potato/onion mix on bottom of greased pan.

Layer on ½ of soup and cheese.

Repeat steps 3 and 4 with remaining ingredients.

Bake for 2 hours.

Serve.

7. Which of the following is the first step enumerated in the process of making scalloped potatoes?
   A. Slice ½ pound potatoes.
   B. Roughly chop onions.
   C. Preheat the oven.
   D. Mix potatoes and onions.

Registration Steps for Community College

Please submit the admissions application. This must be done prior to registering for classes.

Once accepted, look at the schedule of classes.

Be sure to check all course prerequisites.

Class registration steps

First, log in to MyDCC.

Next, click on Class Registration.

Then, click on the relevant registration term.

Choose the courses. Click on each course you wish to take.

Finally, click Register.

Print your schedule.

Pay your fees and tuition online before the deadline.

Buy your books online (at MyBooks.com) or in person at the Student Union bookstore.

Questions?

If help is needed after attempting the process on MyDCC, please call (555) 555-9924 or email DCCregistration@edu.org.

8. According to the registration steps, what is the first action that must be completed?
   A. Pay fees and tuition online.
   B. Call or email.
   C. Log into MyDCC.
   D. Submit an admissions application.

1. Imagine three colored marbles in a jar; one is red and two are blue.
2. Remove a blue marble.
3. Add a yellow marble.
4. Add a red marble.
5. Remove a blue marble.
6. Add a yellow marble.

9. Which of the following is the number of marbles of each color the jar now contains?
   A. 2 red, 2 yellow
   B. 2 blue, 2 yellow
   C. 2 red, 1 blue, 1 yellow
   D. 2 yellow, 1 red, 1 blue

10. Start with the shape pictured below. Follow the directions to alter its appearance.

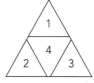

1. Draw a circle that completely encloses the shape.
2. Remove section 1 from the shape.
3. Remove section 3 from the shape.
4. Replace section 1 onto the shape, in its original spot.
5. Remove section 2 from the shape.

Which of the following does the shape now look like?

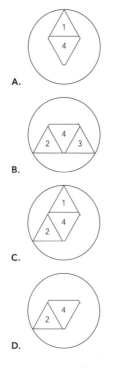

A.

B.

C.

D.

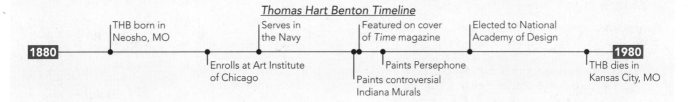

Thomas Hart Benton Timeline

THB born in Neosho, MO
1880
Serves in the Navy
Enrolls at Art Institute of Chicago
Featured on cover of *Time* magazine
Paints Persephone
Paints controversial Indiana Murals
Elected to National Academy of Design
1980
THB dies in Kansas City, MO

11. Which of the following statements is accurate based on the timeline?
   A. Thomas Hart Benton was born in Kansas City.
   B. Immediately after enrolling at the Art Institute of Chicago, Thomas Hart Benton served in the Navy.
   C. The controversy over the Indiana Murals landed Thomas Hart Benton on the cover of *Time* magazine.
   D. Thomas Hart Benton died in the 1970s.

12. A young boy has an allergy to all types of nuts. Which of the following candy bars is safe for him?
   A. Indulge Bar – Ingredients: dark chocolate, cocoa butter, skim milk, corn syrup, sugar, soy protein, peanut butter, artificial flavor
   B. Chocolate Extreme – Ingredients: milk chocolate, cocoa butter, raisins, skim milk, corn syrup, chopped pecans, sugar, soy protein, artificial flavor
   C. Vanilla Blast – Ingredients: white chocolate, whey protein, skim milk, vanilla flavor, almond extract, corn syrup, sugar, soy protein
   D. Chocolate Crunch – Ingredients: milk chocolate, rice puffs, skim milk, corn syrup, sugar, soy protein, malt powder, soybean oil, artificial flavor

Three candidates showed up for an interview. Of all the candidates, only one was appropriate for the job. The first candidate arrived promptly and was dressed professionally. She spoke articulately and seemed a good fit for the organization. The next candidate was also on time, but his dress shirt was stained, his tie was crooked, and he seemed to struggle with the standard interview questions. His performance during the interview was not as impressive as the first candidate's performance. The final candidate, dressed in a T-shirt and ripped jeans, arrived a full hour past the scheduled interview time. Because of her tardiness, we did not interview her.

13. Which of the following is the author's overall conclusion concerning the second candidate?
   A. The stain on the second candidate's shirt distracted the interviewer.
   B. The second candidate was sloppily dressed.
   C. The second candidate had an unimpressive interview performance.
   D. The second candidate was late to the interview.

14. Which of the following sentences would be a supporting detail for an advertisement's claim that a given company provides "industry-leading customer service"?
   A. Our call response times are proven to be 50% faster than our competitors.
   B. We sell products made from only the highest-quality materials.
   C. None of our competitors can match our incredibly low prices.
   D. Our customer service is second to none.

The next two questions are based on this memo.

Debra –

I just heard about the new executive opening. It seems a little unusual to add new people there, especially when some of the other departments need staff.

All that to the side, I think you should consider Alex Jones from Accounting. I think his skills are wasted at his current job; he would make an excellent manager. He's done everything we asked him to, and more. Everyone down here likes him, and I can't imagine him doing anything to disappoint you – or the company, for that matter. Just call him up for an interview, and I think you'll see what I mean.

Also, we're getting Chinese food delivered later, so give any menu requests to Andy.

Regards,

Hal

15. Which of the following best captures the author's purpose?
   A. Ensure another person is not hired for an executive position
   B. Ensure all departments are equally staffed
   C. Get Alex Jones an interview for the open executive position
   D. Ensure everyone gets Chinese for dinner

16. Which of the following most likely describes the relationship between the director of human resources and the employee?
   A. Friendship
   B. Fear
   C. Hostility and anger
   D. Familiarity and trust

The next two questions are based on this passage.

Going one-to-one with computers and students in middle school is a waste of money and teachers' time. Students in middle school are too young to manage the independent use of computers. A recent study shows that 75% of middle school-age teens spend, on average, 5 hours per day on social media. This does not allow for enough hours in a day for academics. There will be more problems with keeping students off of social media and focused on academic endeavors, such as reading in print, practicing "drill and kill" math, and reading social studies textbook chapters. After all, there is plenty of time in high school for students to apply 21st-century skills, such as computer usage.

17. Which of the following methods of argument is used in the previous passage?
   A. Analogy
   B. Attack of an opposing argument
   C. Specific evidence
   D. Emotional argument

18. Which of the following statements would weaken the argument?
   A. Recent high scores on an online, standardized test taken by middle school students
   B. Various types of social media
   C. Examples of teachers who do not know how to use computers for academic purposes
   D. Demonstration why social media cannot be used in a classroom.

Jermaine was a debate champion *par excellence*. He never became flustered; he always had a ready response. His introductions and conclusions were both concise and precise. Indeed, he had a well-deserved reputation for spouting *mots justes*.

19. The use of italics in the text signifies which of the following?
   A. Foreign phrases
   B. Emphasized words
   C. References to footnotes
   D. Words used in unconventional ways

20. Which of the following would be a primary source for a paper about a famous author?
   A. A review of one of the author's books
   B. The author's personal correspondence
   C. An encyclopedia entry about the author
   D. A biography written about the author

Store	Shipping and Handling
Janitor Depot	$30 total for any order
Hyperion Cleaning Supplies	$40 total for any order
Southern Cleaning and Maintenance	$30 for orders less than $100; free for orders $100 or more
Maid Central	$2 per case

21. A company wants to buy 10 cases of cleaning fluid at $10 per case. Based on the pricing chart, which of the following stores will provide the least expensive shipping and handling for this order?
   A. Janitor Depot
   B. Hyperion Cleaning Supplies
   C. Southern Cleaning and Maintenance
   D. Maid Central

22. An aspiring author wants to be sure that her novel is properly formatted and wants to avoid making errors of which her English teacher would disapprove. Which of the following resources is most appropriate in this case?
   A. *The Philadelphia Manual of Grammar Style*
   B. *How to Plot a Breakthrough Novel*
   C. *New Literary Horizons: A Journal of Contemporary Fiction*
   D. The personal website of author Kevin Handel

The next two questions are based on this passage.

A well-known Midwestern publishing company has estimated that 80,000 to 100,000 people in the United States want a collection of anti-war song lyrics from the 1970s. What accounts for this renewed interest in the 70s songs? As studies show, the engaging anti-war sentiments impact a politically involved audience.

23. Which of the following statements best supports the argument in this paragraph?
   A. Anti-war song lyrics are more interesting than song lyrics today.
   B. People today are politically involved and relate to the messages in anti-war lyrics.
   C. Publishing companies are putting together a collection of 1970s song lyrics.
   D. Midwesterners have a renewed interested in 1970s lyrics.

24. Which of the following additional sentences would be expected for this passage if the theme were being addressed by a military publication?
   A. How those sentiments influence policy decisions is an open question that bears careful scrutiny.
   B. Focusing the energy behind those sentiments into a concerted movement is the ultimate goal.
   C. A more politically involved culture will ultimately lead to a decrease in military spending.
   D. The research indicates an opportunity for new artists to gain popularity through political messages.

The next six questions are based on this passage.

Mr. Grundle's New Leaf Blower

Mr. Grundle purchased a new leaf blower and set the box out in his yard. He attempted to pull open the heavy packaging with his hands, but failed. Then he brought scissors, but the heavy material proved too tough for him. Finally he decided to bring out a hacksaw. When he was finished, the box lay in tatters all across the lawn. After the mess was cleaned up, Mr. Grundle set to work with his new purchase. He strapped the blower on his back, aimed at a leaf pile, and pulled the trigger. Nothing happened. He removed the leaf blower and began a 20-minute examination of the device. Finally he decided that he should probably add gasoline. Ten minutes later, Mr. Grundle's driveway was a river of spilled gasoline. He did manage to get a bit of it into the leaf blower, though. Finally he got the gasoline cleaned up and the leaf blower strapped onto his back again. It was time for another try. This time the device roared to life, and leaves went flying every which way. Mr. Grundle was initially pleased with the effect, but less so when he noticed that the leaves were hard to control. They blew and scattered all across the lawn; he needed to be more careful about where he aimed. Finally, after pushing leaves around for half an hour and making a bigger mess than he started with, Mr. Grundle finally began to get the hang of his new machine. Unfortunately, at that very moment the blower ran out of gas. Mr. Grundle took the blower into his garage, emerged with a rake, and proceeded to rake his lawn. The next day, neighbors were surprised to see a shiny new leaf blower sitting in his trashcan.

25. Which of the following provides the best summary of the passage?
    A. Mr. Grundle threw his leaf blower in the trash after it caused him trouble. When he tried to fill it with gasoline, the gasoline spilled all over his driveway and he had to spend time cleaning up his mess before he could use his leaf blower. There was a river of gasoline in his driveway!
    B. Mr. Grundle purchased a new leaf blower, and after struggling to open it, finally strapped it on and found that it didn't work because it needed gas. After cleaning up the gasoline mess he made in his driveway, Mr. Grundle tried his leaf blower again, but found it difficult to control the leaves. He eventually gave up, raked his leaves instead, and threw his new leaf blower in the trash.
    C. Mr. Grundle purchased a new leaf blower and put the box out in his yard so that he could open it up. He tried first to open it with his bare hands. Then, he tried using scissors but that didn't work. Eventually, he used a hacksaw to open the box, which made a huge mess that he had to clean up before he could use his new leaf blower.
    D. Mr. Grundle found his new leaf blower difficult to use. Even when he tried to be careful, it blew his leaves all over his yard and made a bigger mess than if he had not used the leaf blower at all. He eventually gave up and raked his leaves instead.

26. Which of the following is the most likely reason the neighbors saw Mr. Grundle's leaf blower in the trashcan?
    A. Mr. Grundle was out of gas for his new leaf blower.
    B. The leaf blower was too powerful for Mr. Grundle's small yard.
    C. Mr. Grundle determined that it was easier to rake his leaves than use his new leaf blower.
    D. The leaf blower did not turn on when Mr. Grundle pulled the trigger.

27. Which of the following could be considered the main idea of this passage?
    A. Gasoline, hacksaws, and leaves all make messes that homeowners must clean up.
    B. Rakes are more useful than leaf blowers.
    C. Always read the instructions before powering on a new device.
    D. Sometimes tools intended to make a job easier actually make a job more difficult.

28. Which of the following lists Mr. Grundle's actions in the correct sequence?
    A. Mr. Grundle purchased a new leaf blower, made a mess of his yard by blowing the leaves everywhere, and then decided to rake his leaves instead.
    B. Mr. Grundle raked his leaves and then decided to purchase a new leaf blower, which he filled with gasoline that spilled all over his driveway.
    C. Mr. Grundle used a hacksaw to open his new leaf blower, and then had to use scissors to open the rest of the packaging.
    D. Mr. Grundle pulled his new leaf blower from the box and carefully examined it before strapping it on, aiming at a leaf pile, and pulling the trigger.

29. The passage states that after trying to fill his leaf blower with fuel, "Mr. Grundle's driveway was a river of spilled gasoline." Which of the following is the most accurate interpretation of this sentence?
    A. Mr. Grundle lived on a dirty river that was polluted with gasoline.
    B. Mr. Grundle had spilled a large amount of gasoline in his driveway that seemed to be flowing much like a river would.
    C. Mr. Grundle spilled a small amount of gasoline in his driveway.
    D. Mr. Grundle's driveway was near a river that smelled like gasoline.

30. Which of the following statements based on the passage should be considered an opinion?
    A. Mr. Grundle should have been more patient in figuring out how to use his new leaf blower.
    B. After struggling to remove the packaging, Mr. Grundle hacked it to pieces.
    C. By the time Mr. Grundle mastered the use of his leaf blower, it ran out of gas.
    D. Mr. Grundle surprised his neighbors by throwing the leaf blower into the trash.

The next three questions are based on this passage.

Dear Team,

The time has come to select your office space in our new building, which should be move-in ready by the end of the month! We will be selecting our spaces by seniority. For your convenience, I've listed names below by employment tenure. The official map-recorder is Mary, and she will record your desired space on her master map at the front desk. When it is your time to select a space, Mary will notify you. We ask that you spend some time reviewing the map now so that when the time comes to select your space, you can do so quickly. We hope to have this process completed within two days.

As always, if you have any questions, please notify me. Happy space-hunting!

Jerry

Office space selection order

1. Mary	5. Rachel	9. Darius	13. Luis
2. Vincent	6. Jerry	10. Connie	14. Shonda
3. Sonia	7. Juanita	11. Phil	15. Claire
4. Misha	8. Shelly	12. Shelby	

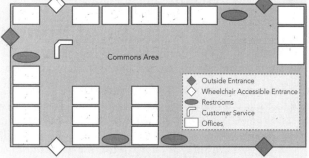

31. Based on information included on the map of the building, which of the following is the number of entrances in the building?
    A. Two
    B. Three
    C. Four
    D. Five

32. Which of the following text features from Jerry's message is used to assist with a process?
    A. Map legend
    B. Bolded words "end of the month"
    C. Numbered list of employees by seniority
    D. Underlined words "2 days"

33. Assuming that everyone on the list selects an office space, which of the following is the number of spaces that will be left unoccupied in the new building?
    A. 1
    B. 2
    C. 3
    D. 4

The next two questions are based on this passage.

Do you want to increase your IQ dramatically in just one short month? Become smarter by following my simple brain-energizing program. This program includes daily mental exercises, nutrition and fitness guides, and daily vitamin and nutrient supplements, all of which will help boost your IQ. With five easy payments of $19.99, we can guarantee that you will impress your friends and family with your newfound intelligence in just four weeks.

34. Which of the following choices is part of this brain-energizing program?
    A. Calendar and payment envelopes
    B. Vitamins and mental exercises
    C. IQ test and written guarantee
    D. Intelligence and friends

35. Which of the following best describes the author's purpose?
    A. He wants to impress his friends and family.
    B. He wants to sell his brain-energizing program and make a profit.
    C. He wants to increase the average IQ score of people across the country.
    D. He wants to improve the health of his customers.

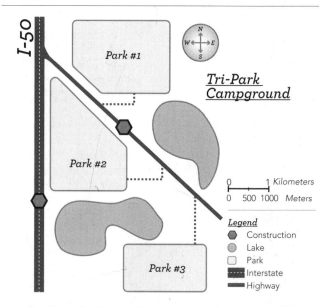

36. A family is driving via Interstate 50. They are traveling from south to north. If the family visits all three parks on the map, and then turns around and drives back home using the same route, which of the following indicates the number of times their car will pass through a possible roadblock?
    A. 1
    B. 2
    C. 3
    D. 4

37. The diagram represents a blood pressure monitor. Which of the following indicates the diastolic blood pressure reading?

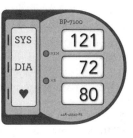

A. 72
B. 80
C. 121
D. 152

38. Which of the following sentences indicates the start of a sequence?
A. The foremost thought in my mind is that we keep the project on schedule.
B. Finally, we headed to the airport to catch our flight.
C. I first grabbed a bite to eat at my favorite dinner spot.
D. We immediately headed downtown to meet our contact.

The pitcher slouched over, hands on his knees, and spit in the dirt as the batter jauntily rounded the bases. The game was suddenly close again, and the tall lefty looked over to his team's dugout and saw the manager emerging.

39. Which of the following conclusions is well supported by the passage?
A. The baseball game is nearly over.
B. The pitcher's team is going to lose.
C. The batter has hit a home run.
D. The manager is tall.

The next two questions are based on this passage.

The obstacle course first requires that athletes jump through three tires, which are suspended from ropes attached to the ceiling of the gymnasium. Then, after skateboarding around a series of large orange cones, participants must strap a heavy sandbag weight to their backs and scale a 10-foot wall. If they make it over that obstacle, they are almost certain to complete the course successfully – unless eating live worms is a problem.

40. Which of the following best describes the structure of this text?
A. Compare/contrast
B. Problem/solution
C. Sequence
D. Cause/effect

41. Based on the context, which of the following is the meaning of the word "scale" in the passage?
A. Musical pitches played in an ascending or descending regular interval
B. Instrument used to weigh things
C. A part of a fish's skin
D. Climb up and over

The next two questions are based on this passage.

Dear Sean,

Congratulations on winning the State High School Football Player of the Year award. It is an incredible accomplishment – one that you will treasure forever. Your tremendous motivational drive and superior athletic skills were apparent to us right from the start, and we are tremendously pleased that the award voters saw exactly what we saw in you.

Looking ahead, we can see even greater things in your future. Your choice of college will have a profound effect on exactly how great those things are – so we hope you're still planning to visit our campus this spring. We have a fun day of activities planned for you. By the time it's done, we think you'll agree that Eastern Reserve University is the perfect place to continue your winning tradition.

Best Regards,

Bill Meehan, Athletic Director
Eastern Reserve University

42. Which of the following statements from the passage is a fact?
A. Sean will forever treasure his title as State High School Football Player of the Year.
B. Sean is the State High School Football Player of the Year.
C. We have a fun day of activities planned for you.
D. Eastern Reserve University is the perfect place for Sean to continue his schooling.

43. Which of the following statements best describes the author's point of view?
A. Motivational drive and superior athletic skills are important qualities for a person to have.
B. Sean is a talented athlete and should attend Eastern Reserve University to play football.
C. Sean is proud of winning State High School Football Player of the Year.
D. It is important to plan ahead and select a university early.

She is a gregarious individual who can always be found laughing with friends.

44. Which of the following is the meaning of "gregarious" as used in the sentence?
A. High-spirited
B. Energetic
C. Inquisitive
D. Sociable

Carbon, 254, 559-64, 670

Cesium, 271, 655-6

Chrome, 219

Chromium, 220

Chromium alloys, 221-2, 503

Chromium oxidation, 223-4

45. A chemistry student wants to learn about a chromium alloy. Using the excerpt from a science textbook's index, on which of the following pages should the student begin to look?

A. 219
B. 220
C. 221
D. 223

Chapter 2: The Dinosaurs

1. Where They Lived

   A. Africa

   B. Asia

   C. Australia

   D. _____

   E. North America

2. When They Lived

3. What They Ate

46. Examine the headings. Based on the pattern, which of the following is a reasonable heading to insert in the blank spot?

A. China
B. Europe
C. Mexico
D. Middle East

47. A customer at an electronics store is describing to a salesperson the ideal computer for her. The following is a list of the customer's criteria.

· Dual-core processor

· Dedicated graphics system

· Minimum 400 gigabyte hard drive

· G speed wireless connectivity

Which of the following is an appropriate choice for this customer?

A.

Processor	2.5 GHz dual core
Graphics Subsystem	Dedicated
Front-Side Bus	800 ghz
Hard Drive	800 gigabytes
Memory	6 gigabytes
Connectivity	Wireless G, optional cellular modem

B.

Processor	3 GHz dual core
Graphics Subsystem	Dedicated
Front-Side Bus	800 ghz
Hard Drive	750 gigabytes
Memory	4 gigabytes
Connectivity	Wireless B, optional cellular modem

C.

Processor	2.5 GHz dual core
Graphics Subsystem	Dedicated
Front-Side Bus	600 ghz
Hard Drive	350 gigabytes
Memory	4 gigabytes
Connectivity	Wireless G, optional cellular modem

D.

Processor	3 GHz single core
Graphics Subsystem	Dedicated
Front-Side Bus	600 ghz
Hard Drive	750 gigabytes
Memory	6 gigabytes
Connectivity	Wireless G, optional cellular modem

Reading section quiz rationales

1. Option B is correct. This summary sentence defines the topic and briefly explains the effect. Option A only addresses one result of this option. It does not define the topic (call options) nor address the negative possibilities. Option B doesn't summarize the overall information in the passage. Although the author points out the complexity of call options, the passage is focused on examples of how they function. Option D makes a generalization that is not substantiated with supporting key ideas. See R.1.1 for related information.

2. Option C is correct. The statement "Call options allowed her to bet on the market without taking on too much risk" implies that investors should be aware of this option. Therefore, a conclusion can be drawn about the low-risk opportunity. Option A is an explanation of a call option but is not a conclusion. A conclusion is a message the reader draws from the text. Each case shows Option B as effects of investing. However, it is not the overall message the author is implying. Ultimately, Sharon's purchase is only an example, and Option D is not the message of the informative passage. See R.1.2 for related information.

3. Option C is correct. This definition is explicitly and specifically stated. See R.1.5 for related information.

4. Option D is correct. According to the example paragraph, Sharon reacts to her belief that stock XYZ will go up. She buys call options. Then, a month later, she takes action. See R.1.7 for related information.

5. Option A is correct. This passage explains what a call option is and gives examples to clarify. This passage does not form a visual or use sensory details. Rhetorical, persuasive language is not used to sway; rather, the passage just informs. This passage does not tell a story, use sensory details, or demonstrate chronological order. See R.2.2 for related information.

6. Option B is correct. The context clue here is "only a few understand stock options." The author uses case study to show diverse results. There is subtle description, but the majority of the passage is to inform. There are case studies, or anecdotes, in this passage. However, they are not considered stories, and the passage does not contain literary elements. The author is not persuading the reader to purchase call options; rather, the author is informing the reader on how to purchase and why. The author describes call options, but the remainder of the passage informs the reader on results of diverse actions. See R.2.5 for related information.

7. Option C is correct. The first step is found under the subhead steps and numbered 1. See R.1.4 for related information.

8. Option D is correct. Even though the signal words first, next, then, and finally appear in step 3, the first step is to compete the admissions application. It is No. 1 and mentions that nothing can be done until this step is complete. Option A cannot be done until student is accepted and registered. The phone number and email are only for people who have attempted the process on MyDCC. Option D is the first step in the third action. See R.1.4 for related information.

9. Option A is correct. Following the directions produces the following results: 1. Jar contents: 1 red, 2 blue; 2. 1 red, 1 blue; 3. 1 red, 1 blue, 1 yellow; 4. 2 red, 1 blue, 1 yellow; 5. 2 red, 1 yellow; 6. 2 red, 2 yellow. See R.1.4 for related information.

10. Option A is correct. See R.1.4 for related information.

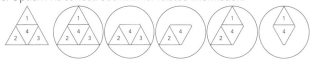

11. Option D is correct. The proximity of this information on the timeline to the end date of 1980 indicates that is accurate. The timeline indicates that Thomas Hart Benton was born in Neosho, Missouri. The space between Option B events on the timeline indicates that one did not occur immediately after the other. The timeline does not indicate causality between Option C events. See R.1.6 for related information.

12. Option D is correct. This is the only list of ingredients that does not include nuts of any kind or in any form. Peanut butter is included on the ingredient list for Option A. Chopped pecans are included on the ingredient list for Option B. Almond extract is included on the ingredient list for Option C. See R.1.5 for related information.

13. Option C is correct. His sloppy dress, tardiness, and struggle with interview questions made for an unimpressive performance. See R.1.2 for related information.

14. Option A is correct. Response times are directly related to customer service, so this statement supports the idea of industry-leading customer service. Options B and C are not directly related to customer service. Option D is a restatement of the claim, not a supporting detail. See R.1.3 for related information.

15. Option C is correct. The author uses persuasive speech and detail to ensure the director is aware of Alex Jones' strengths for the specific position. The author uses a paragraph to persuade the director to consider interviewing another employee for the executive opening. Even though the author mentions other departments needing staff, the remainder of the email encourages the director to hire Alex Jones. The menu requests are mentioned last. Ordering Chinese food is a reminder, not the purpose of the email. See R.2.5 for related information.

16. Option D is correct. The employee uses very persuasive and educated statements, such as "It seems a little unusual to add new people there, especially when some of the other departments need staff." There is apparent trust because of the employee's willingness to challenge and recommend. However, there is no evidence of personal discussion, which would demonstrate friendship. It is clear that the employee is not fearful because he not only questions the director's motives, but also makes a recommendation. There is no angry or hostile word choice. In fact, the employee ends with a reminder about a group lunch. See R.3.2 for related information.

17. Option C is correct. This passage shares specific evidence that middle school-aged teenagers spend a lot of time on social media. There is not an analogy in this passage. This passage does not attack an opposition, and there are no signal words that move the passage into an opposing argument. This paragraph is strictly expository. Its diction is noncommittal and factual. See R.2.1 for related information.

18. Option A is correct. This would be an argument used by an opposing side. It would weaken the idea that middle school students cannot focus on academics online. See R.3.4 for related information.

19. Option A is correct. A reader familiar with the convention of italicizing foreign words should understand that the words italicized here are not English, even if the actual meaning of those words is not understood. See R.2.7 for related information.

20. Option B is correct. Letters written by the author are a primary source. Option A is a secondary source because it interprets the primary source, which is the book itself. Options C and D are secondary sources because they interpret the primary source, which is the author's life. See R.3.1 for related information.

21. Option C is correct. Southern Cleaning and Maintenance's free shipping rate for orders more than $100 makes it the least expensive shipping option. Janitor Depot would charge $30 for shipping and handling. Hyperion Cleaning Supplies would charge $40 for shipping and handling. Maid Central would charge $20 to ship 10 cases. See R.3.5 for related information.

22. Option A is correct. The author's goals are to format the novel correctly and to avoid basic English errors. A manual of grammar and style is an appropriate choice, as it likely covers these topics. See R.3.1 for related information.

23. Option B is correct. This statement supports the argument because the message of the paragraph discusses the engagement with the lyrics due to the political sentiments. See R.3.4 for related information.

24. Option A is correct. A military publication would likely be interested in how anti-war sentiments could affect policy that could, in turn, affect military operations. Option B would be expected from an anti-war publication. Option C is not supported by the evidence presented and is not an idea that a military publication would likely advance. Option D is not an angle on which a military publication would likely focus. See R.3.3 for related information.

25. Option B is correct. This option offers the most complete summary. It includes a sequential retelling of the most important details. Option A focuses too much on the gas spill and does not include all of the important details from the passage. Option C focuses too much on the purchasing and opening up of the leaf blower. It does not include all of the important details from the passage. Option D leaves out many of the challenges Mr. Grundle faced, as well as the fact that he eventually threw away his leaf blower. See R.1.1 for related information.

26. Option C is correct. Based on the difficulties Mr. Grundle had with his leaf blower, and the fact that he ultimately put down his leaf blower and raked his leaves instead, this is the most likely explanation. His leaf blower ran out of gas, but he could have refilled it. The passage does not say anything about his yard being small. Although the leaves went everywhere, that was most likely because Mr. Grundle was not yet skilled at using the leaf blower. The leaf blower did not initially turn on when Mr. Grundle pulled the trigger because he had failed to put gas in it. See R.1.2 for related information.

27. Option D is correct. This is the main idea communicated by the passage. See R.1.3 for related information.

28. Option A is correct. This is the order in which the events of the story occur. Mr. Grundle raked his leaves only after he became frustrated with his new leaf blower. Mr. Grundle tried using scissors first, and then resorted to using a hacksaw. Mr. Grundle examined the leaf blower carefully only after he pulled the trigger and found that it didn't work. See R.1.7 for related information.

29. Option B is correct. Given the context, this is clearly the correct answer. The passage does not suggest that Mr. Grundle lived on a river. The "river of spilled gasoline" would not be a small amount of gasoline. See R.2.3 for related information.

30. Option A is correct. The key word "should" indicates a value judgment and an opinion. Options B, C, and D are supported by the details of the passage and do not contain opinion. See R.2.1 for related information.

31. Option D is correct. There are five entrances total, including those that are wheelchair-accessible. There are two wheelchair-accessible entrances, three outside entrances, and four restrooms. See R.1.6 for related information.

32. Option C is correct. This list serves to organize the employees so that they will follow the process of selecting spaces in order of seniority. Option A informs the employees about the layout of the building, but does not contribute to the process of office space selection that the employees are expected to follow. Option B emphasizes the time of the move, but does not assist with the process of selecting spaces. Option D emphasizes the timeline, but does not assist with the process of selecting spaces. See R.2.7 for related information.

33. Option D is correct. There are 19 spaces and 15 employees needing to select spaces, which leaves four spaces unoccupied. See R.3.5 for related information.

34. Option B is correct. These are listed in the description as part of the program. There is no mention of a calendar or payment envelopes. The writer does not state that there is a written guarantee, nor an IQ test. The program itself does not come with intelligence or friends. See R.1.5 for related information.

35. Option B is correct. The author tells customers to "become smarter by following" his program, and tells them they can have it for only "five easy payments of $19.99." The author's primary goal is to sell the product. See R.2.5 for related information.

36. Option D is correct. Following the route described, the family's car will pass through each of the two possible roadblocks twice, for a total of four times. See R.1.6 for related information.

37. Option A is correct. Even if the meaning of diastolic blood pressure or how it is measured is unknown, clues are provided on the device. In this case, DIA represents diastolic measurement, which is 72. Option B is the heart rate, as indicated by the heart-shaped symbol that corresponds with the number 80. Option C is the systolic measurement, as indicated by the abbreviation SYS that corresponds with the number 121. Option D is the sum of the systolic measurement and the heart rate. See R.1.6 for related information.

38. Option C is correct. The keyword "first" indicates that additional events following this one will be described. While Option A mentions a project, it does not provide any indication about how this action relates to sequence. The key word "finally" indicates that Option B occurs later in a sequence. Option D does not provide any indicate about how this action relates to sequence. See R.1.7 for related information.

39. Option C is correct. This conclusion is supported by the fact that the batter is "jauntily" running around all the bases. There is no information in the passage about the point at which this action occurs during the game. The passage indicates that the game is close, so it's impossible to say which team will win or lose. The description "tall lefty" refers to the pitcher. See R.1.2 for related information.

40. Option C is correct. The author tells in sequential order what participants will encounter as they race through the obstacle course. The passage does not compare or contrast two or more entities. The obstacle course is not characterized as a problem in need of a solution. There is no cause or effect in this passage. See R.2.2 for related information.

41. Option D is correct. In this context, scale is a verb. Participants will climb up and over a 10-foot wall. See R.2.3 for related information.

42. Option B is correct. This is a fact because it can be verified as being a true statement. See R.2.1 for related information.

43. Option B is correct. This most accurately describes the author's point of view. Sean is not the author of this passage. There is no indication that Mr. Meehan believes Option D to be true. See R.2.6 for related information.

44. Option D is correct. An individual who is gregarious enjoys the companionship of others and can be viewed as sociable. See R.2.4 for related information.

45. Option C is correct. According to the textbook's index, the first relevant entry regarding information about chromium alloys can be found on pages 221 and 222. You could find information on chrome on page 219. You could find information on chromium on page 220, but the index does not mention the alloy in the description. There is a more relevant series of pages. You could find information about chromium oxidation starting on page 223. See R.3.1 for related information.

46. Option B is correct. The existing headings establish a definite pattern of continents. Of the available options, Europe is the only continent. See R.3.1 for related information.

47. Option A is correct. This is the only option that meets all the customer's criteria. These computer terms and numbers might mean nothing to some readers, but the answer can be discovered even without any knowledge of computers. The correct answer is revealed through a process of elimination. Option B does not have wireless G connectivity. Option C does not have enough gigabytes for the hard drive. Option D does not have a dual-core processor. See R.3.5 for related information.

Mathematics

The objectives for the Mathematics section of the TEAS are organized in two categories.

Number and algebra (M.1)   *23 questions*

M.1.1. Convert among non-negative fractions, decimals, and percentages.
M.1.2. Perform arithmetic operations with rational numbers.
M.1.3. Compare and order rational numbers.
M.1.4. Solve equations in one variable.
M.1.5. Solve real-world one- or multi-step problems with rational numbers.
M.1.6. Solve real-world problems involving percentages.
M.1.7. Apply estimation strategies and rounding rules to real-world problems.
M.1.8. Solve real-world problems involving proportions.
M.1.9. Solve real-world problems involving ratios and rates of change.
M.1.10. Translate phrases and sentences into expressions, equations, and inequalities.

Measurement and data (M.2)   *9 questions*

M.2.1. Interpret relevant information from tables, charts, and graphs.
M.2.2. Evaluate the information in tables, charts, and graphs using statistics.
M.2.3. Explain the relationship between two variables.
M.2.4. Calculate geometric quantities.
M.2.5. Convert within and between standard and metric systems.

Remember, there are 32 scored Mathematics items on the TEAS. These are divided as shown above. In addition, there will be four unscored pretest items that can be in any of these categories.

M.1.1 *Convert among non-negative fractions, decimals, and percentages.*

Number quantities can be represented in many ways, including fractions, decimals, and percentages. For this task on the TEAS, you'll need to understand each of these forms and how to convert between them. You should practice converting from one number quantity to another until you've mastered the processes. There are plenty of exercises available on the Internet for honing your skill at converting among number quantities, and the overview below will provide the base of knowledge you'll need to succeed at this task.

A fraction is a numeric expression dividing one number by another. Fractions can be written in the form a/b or $\frac{a}{b}$, where a and b are integers. The a (the first or top integer) is the numerator, and the b (the second or bottom integer) is the denominator. The value of a fraction is found by dividing the numerator by the denominator.

As an example, ⅗ or $\frac{3}{5}$ is three-fifths, or three parts (portion) out of five parts (the whole thing). To find the value, divide numerator 3 by denominator 5 (3 into calculator first, then "/", then 5). You get a decimal value of 0.6. This illustrates how to convert from a fraction to a decimal.

Another form of number quantity is decimal form. Numbers in decimal form have place values, some of which are illustrated by the following chart.

The number 3,452.68 is read "three thousand, four hundred fifty-two and sixty-eight hundredths." The decimal number 0.00087 is read "eighty-seven hundred thousandths." The decimal part of any number can be read ending with the decimal place of the last non-zero digit. In the case of 0.00087, the 7 is the last non-zero decimal digit. Because the 7 is in the "hundred thousandths" place, this is how it is expressed.

To convert from decimal to fraction form, there are a couple of scenarios to consider: a value greater than 1, and a value less than 1.

If a decimal value is greater than 1, for example 2.36, move the decimal to the right until you have a whole number (in this case, 236). Keep track of how many decimal places you moved the decimal. This whole number becomes the numerator. Then, your denominator becomes a 1 followed by the number of zeros that matches the number of places the decimal moved (2.36 to 236 implies the decimal moved to the right two places). The denominator becomes a 1 followed two zeros (100). The fraction representation of 2.36 is thus $\frac{236}{100}$. If the decimal was 2.036, move the decimal to the right until you have a whole number (in this case, 2036), and keep track of how many decimal places you moved the decimal. This whole number becomes the numerator. Then, your denominator becomes a 1 followed by the number of zeros that match the number of places the decimal moved (2.036 to 2036 means the decimal moved to the right three places). The denominator becomes a 1 followed by three zeros (1,000). The fraction representation of 2.036 is thus $\frac{2036}{1000}$. You can also try to simplify, or reduce, fractions if possible.

This objective includes, but is not limited to, the following examples of knowledge, skills, and abilities.

- *Know the relationship between the numerator and denominator in a fraction.*
- *Demonstrate knowledge of place value within decimals.*
- *Define percent as a number out of 100.*

Key terms

decimal. A number expressed in powers of 10.

denominator. The bottom number of a fraction.

fraction. A number expressed as a numerator and denominator.

integer. Whole numbers and their negatives: …, -3, -2, -1, 0, 1, 2, 3, …

non-negative. Greater than or equal to zero (positive or zero).

numerator. The top number of a fraction.

percent. Parts per hundred.

place value. Numerical value defined by position.

whole number. The numbers used in counting and zero: 0, 1, 2, 3, 4, 5, 6, 7, …

MATHEMATICS

If a decimal value is less than 1, for example 0.36, simply use 36 as the numerator, and the place value of the last decimal digit as the denominator (in this case, hundredths). The decimal 0.36 would be written as $\frac{36}{100}$, and read thirty-six hundredths. If the decimal was 0.036, it would be written as $\frac{36}{1000}$, and read thirty-six thousandths.

Percent is a third form of number quantity. Percent means "per 100", or a value's proportional equivalent compared to 100. One percent can be interpreted as one one-hundredth ($\frac{1}{100}$) of something. Examples of percent expressions are 45%, 23.8%, 100%, and 0.05%. To convert 45% to a decimal, divide the number by 100 and remove the percent symbol. So, $\frac{45}{100}$ gives 0.45.

A decimal number can be converted to a percent by multiplying it by 100 and adding a percent sign. For example, 0.67 can be multiplied by 100 to give 67, and then add the percent symbol. So 0.67 equals 67%.

To convert a fraction to a percent, one strategy is to convert to decimal form first. Then convert the decimal to a percent.

To convert a percent to a fraction, one strategy is to convert the percent to a decimal. Then convert the decimal to a fraction.

M.1.1 Practice problems

1. Convert each decimal to a percent.

   A. 1.22

   B. 0.384

   Convert each percent to a decimal.

   C. 73.7%

   D. 138%

   Convert each decimal to a fraction.

   E. 0.516

   F. 1.07

   Convert each fraction to a decimal.

   G. $\frac{19}{10}$

   H. $\frac{13}{50}$

2. Which of the following percentages is equivalent to $\frac{8}{5}$?

   A. 1.6%

   B. 160%

   C. 0.625%

   D. 62.5%

3. Which of the following fractions is equivalent to 83.1%?

   A. $\frac{831}{1000}$

   B. $\frac{83.1}{10}$

   C. $\frac{831}{10}$

   D. 0.831

M.1.2 *Perform arithmetic operations with rational numbers.*

Completing basic computations by hand can at times be quicker than using a calculator. Additionally, calculators don't always complete the mathematical order of operations in ways you assume they will. For this TEAS task, you need to be competent doing these types of calculations by hand. You will apply the order of operations—including addition, subtraction, multiplication, and division—and be expected to do so using integers, decimals, fractions, and mixed numbers. Practice makes perfect, so it might be helpful to search the Internet for additional practice problems.

One mnemonic device for the conventions of the mathematical order of operations for basic calculations is PEMDAS (parentheses, exponents, multiplication and division, addition and subtraction). There is some controversy about the use of PEMDAS (details of which can be easily found by an Internet search), but the TEAS will focus on noncontroversial aspects of the order of operations. For the TEAS, the "E" in PEMDAS (exponents) will not be required. However, parentheses, multiplication and division, and addition and subtraction will be required competencies. To successfully execute these operations, you must (in order) follow these rules.

1. First, perform any calculations inside parentheses.

2. Next, perform all multiplications and divisions, completing the operations as they occur from left to right.

3. Finally, perform all addition and subtraction, completing the operations as they occur from left to right.

The following are three basic examples with rationales.

Ex. 1:

$6 + 7 \times 8 = 6 + \mathbf{7 \times 8}$	**Multiply first.**
$= 6 + 56$	**Then add.**
$= 62$	

Ex. 2:

$16 \div 8 - 2 = \mathbf{16 \div 8} - 2$	**Divide first.**
$= 2 - 2$	**Then subtract.**
$= 0$	

Ex. 3:

$(25 - 11) \times 3 = \mathbf{(25 - 11)} \times 3$	**Perform operations in parentheses first.**
$= 14 \times 3$	**Then multiply.**
$= 42$	

This objective includes, but is not limited to, the following examples of knowledge, skills, and abilities.

- *Complete computations with integers using the four basic operations.*
- *Complete computations with decimals using the four basic operations.*
- *Complete computations with fractions and mixed numbers using the four basic operations.*
- *Complete computations involving the order of operations, excluding complex fractions.*

Key terms

addition. Calculation of a total of two or more numbers.

division. Separation of numbers into parts; the inverse of multiplication.

mixed number. A number formed by an integer and a fraction.

multiplication. Addition of a number to itself a specified number of times.

order of operations. The sequence of operations that must be followed to simplify an expression.

subtraction. Removing one number from another; the inverse of addition.

MATHEMATICS

The following are several examples involving multiple steps.

Example: 3 + 6 × (5 + 4) ÷ 3 - 7

Solution:

Step 1:	3 + 6 × **(5 + 4)** ÷ 3 - 7 = 3 + 6 × 9 ÷ 3 - 7	Parentheses
Step 2:	3 + **6 × 9** ÷ 3 - 7 = 3 + 54 ÷ 3 - 7	Multiplication
Step 3:	3 + **54 ÷ 3** - 7 = 3 + 18 - 7	Division
Step 4:	**3 + 18** - 7 = 21 − 7	Addition
Step 5:	21 - 7 = 14	Subtraction

Example: 9 - 5 ÷ (8 - 3) × 2 + 6

Solution:

Step 1:	9 - 5 ÷ **(8 - 3)** × 2 + 6 = 9 - 5 ÷ 5 × 2 + 6	Parentheses
Step 2:	9 - **5 ÷ 5** × 2 + 6 = 9 - 1 × 2 + 6	Division
Step 3:	9 - **1 × 2** + 6 = 9 - 2 + 6	Multiplication
Step 4:	**9 - 2** + 6 = 7 + 6	Subtraction
Step 5:	7 + 6 = 13	Addition

In the last two examples, you will notice that multiplication and division were evaluated from left to right according to rule 2. Similarly, addition and subtraction were evaluated from left to right, according to rule 3.

When two or more operations occur inside a set of parentheses, these operations should be evaluated according to rules 2 and 3. This is done in the example below.

Example: 150 ÷ (6 + 3 × 8) - 5

Solution:

Step 1:	150 ÷ (6 + **3 × 8**) - 5 = 150 ÷ (6 + 24) - 5	Multiplication inside parentheses
Step 2:	150 ÷ **(6 + 24)** - 5 = 150 ÷ 30 - 5	Addition inside parentheses
Step 3:	**150 ÷ 30** - 5 = 5 - 5	Division
Step 4:	5 - 5 = 0	Subtraction

Example: $\dfrac{36 - 6}{12 + 3}$

Solution:

This problem includes a fraction bar (also called a vinculum), which means we must divide the numerator by the denominator. However, we must perform all calculations above and below the fraction bar BEFORE dividing. Thus:	$\dfrac{36 - 6}{12 + 3} = \dfrac{(36 - 6)}{(12 + 3)}$
Evaluating this expression, we get:	$\dfrac{(36 - 6)}{(12 + 3)} = \dfrac{30}{15} = 2$

Extensions of the above example include decimals, fractions, and mixed numbers. With decimals, all processes are identical. With fractions, you might need to find a common denominator or convert fractions to decimals. The same goes for mixed numbers, but you might need to convert to a fraction first. To help prepare for the TEAS, search the Internet for order of operations practice and work on your mastery of these types of problems.

M.1.2 Practice problems

1. Solve the following problems:

    4 + 3 × (9 - 6)

    (12 - 2) ÷ (11-6)

    6 × 5 + 4 ÷ 2 − 2 × 5

    $\dfrac{30 - 3 \times 2}{18 - 24 \div 2}$

2. Which of the following is the correct value of 3 + 2 × 6 – 4?

    A. 32

    B. 10

    C. 11

    D. 26

3. Which of the following is the correct value of the expression below?

    $\dfrac{15 + 2 \times 5}{11 - 24 \div 4}$

    A. 21

    B. 5

    C. ≈ 9.9

M.1.3 *Compare and order rational numbers.*

Rational numbers are those that we see and use every day, decimals and fractions included. What makes rational numbers unique is that those fractions can be written as either terminating or repeating decimals. For instance, 6 can be written as $\frac{12}{2}$ or $\frac{18}{3}$, but we usually see it in its simplified form: 6. Conversely, irrational numbers cannot be written in fraction form (for example, $\sqrt{2}$ and π converted to decimals are not terminating or repeating).

It is important to be able to put rational numbers in numeric order, as well as visualize and predict situations involving ordered quantities. At times, interpreting ordered number inequality statements is useful as well (like equations, but with inequality symbols instead of equal signs). The TEAS test requires you to compare and order rational numbers. Try searching the Internet using any of the glossary terms to find additional explanations and practice problems.

Integers can be written as fractions by simply writing them over 1. For example, –6, 5, and 100 can be written as $\frac{-6}{1}$, $\frac{5}{1}$, and $\frac{100}{1}$. Therefore, –6, 5 and 100 are rational. Numbers that are not rational include $\sqrt{2}$ ($\sqrt{any\ prime\ number}$, for that matter), the natural number e, and π. One thing you need to remember is that any negative number is "smaller" than any positive number. Essentially, if a number is to the left of another number on the number line, it is smaller. All negative numbers are to the left of all positive numbers.

```
←———•——•——•——•——•——•——•——•——•——•——•———→
   -5   -4   -3   -2   -1    0    1    2    3    4    5
```

To put rational numbers in numeric order (either increasing or decreasing), it can be useful to write the numbers as decimals (unless they are already integers, like –2, –1, 0, 1, 2). Once in decimal form, you can write the numbers vertically, lining up the decimals. For example, the numbers 3.245, 3.524, and 0.3245, can be stacked this way.

3.245

3.524

0.3245

The next thing you do is, starting with the highest place (in this case, the ones place), decide which is the largest (or smallest). Let's put them in decreasing order. Therefore, we need to identify and write the largest value. There are two numbers with 3 in the ones place, so we next need to compare the tenths place for these two numbers.

In this case, the largest is 3.524. Then determine the next largest in the same way: 3.245. And continue this process until all are in order. So in decreasing order, the list would be 3.524, 3.245, 0.3245. Increasing order would be the opposite process, so this list would be 0.3245, 3.245, 3.524.

If the numbers are not in decimal form and you're unsure how to order all of them, you can divide the fractions or fraction parts to get them in decimal form. For instance, for $5\frac{2}{7}$, you can divide 2 by 7 to get 0.2857, so the value becomes 5.2857. Now you can compare to other decimal form numbers.

To compare numbers, we use terms like less than (<), less than or equal to (≤), greater than (>), and greater than or equal to (≥). In the decreasing list 3.524, 3.245, 0.3245, we can write 3.524 > 3.245 > 0.3245. Using the increasing list, we can write 0.3245 < 3.245 < 3.524. We can also write inequalities like 0.3245 ≤ 3.245 because 0.3245 is truly less than OR equal to 3.245. Here the qualifying portion is the "or".

This objective includes, but is not limited to, the following examples of knowledge, skills, and abilities.

- *Demonstrate knowledge of the meaning of rational numbers.*
- *Know the terms and symbols for "greater than," "less than," and "equal to."*
- *Order three or more quantities (least to greatest, greatest to least).*
- *Compare two quantities using symbols.*
- *Know place value with decimals.*
- *Rewrite numbers to have a common denominator.*

MATHEMATICS

Key terms

common denominator. In a set of two or more fractions, an integer that is divisible by each denominator. That is, a multiple of all of the denominators.

decimal place value. Powers of ten by position away from the decimal point. Going left: units, tens, hundreds, etc. Going right: tenths, hundredths, thousandths, etc.

inequality symbols. Less than (<), greater than (>), less than or equal to (≤), and greater than or equal to (≥).

irrational number. A real number that cannot be expressed as terminating or repeating decimals.

multiples of a number. A number multiplied by various integers.

ordering numbers. Putting numbers in order of lowest to highest.

rational number. A number that can be expressed as a fraction.

One can also compare fractions and mixed numbers by converting fraction portions to have common denominators if the denominators are different. To find a common denominator, do the following.

1. Find the least common multiple of the denominators (also called the least common denominator).

2. Change each fraction (using equivalent fractions) to make their denominators the same as the least common denominator.

To get the least common denominator, list the multiples of each denominator (multiplying out to about 7 typically works) and find the smallest number that appears in both lists. If we wanted to compare $\frac{1}{4}$, $\frac{1}{5}$, $\frac{1}{10}$, we could find the least common denominator as follows.

- List the **multiples** of each denominator:
  Multiples of **4** are 8, 12, 16, **20**, 24, 28, …
  Multiples of **5** are 10, 15, **20**, 25, 30, 35 …
  Multiples of **10** are **20**, 30, 40, 50, 60, 70 …

- In the list of multiples, you find that 20 is the smallest number appearing in each list.

- Therefore, the **least common denominator** of $\frac{1}{4}$, $\frac{1}{5}$, and $\frac{1}{10}$, is **20**.

So $\frac{1}{4}$ converted to a denominator of 20 is $\frac{5}{20}$ (both numerator and denominator are multiplied by 5 to get a new denominator of 20). Similarly, $\frac{1}{5}$, becomes $\frac{4}{20}$, and $\frac{1}{10}$, becomes $\frac{2}{20}$. Now that we have common denominators, we can order the fractions. Decreasingly, the order is $\frac{5}{20}$, $\frac{4}{20}$, $\frac{2}{20}$. Once there is a common denominator, you only need to compare the numerators.

This method works pretty well for numbers that aren't too big. The TEAS test will stick to numbers you can handle.

M.1.3 Practice problems

1. Write in increasing order: -5, $5\frac{2}{3}$, 0.523.

2. Which of the following is an expression to compare 8.33 and $8\frac{2}{3}$?
   A. $8.33 > 8\frac{2}{3}$
   B. $8\frac{2}{3} \geq 8.33$
   C. $8.33 = 8\frac{2}{3}$
   D. $8\frac{2}{3} \leq 8.33$

3. Which of the following lists the numbers in decreasing order: -2, -0.2, $2\frac{2}{10}$, 2?
   A. -2, -0.2, 2, $2\frac{2}{10}$
   B. $2\frac{2}{10}$, 2, -2, -0.2
   C. -2, 2, -0.2, $2\frac{2}{10}$
   D. $2\frac{2}{10}$, 2, -0.2, -2

M.1.4 *Solve equations in one variable.*

Algebraic equations consist of variables (letters of the alphabet, sometimes raised to a power), constants (numbers), and an equals sign. Solving equations with one variable requires first collecting all variable terms on one side of the equals sign and all constants on the other side, using addition and/or subtraction. Once all like terms have been combined, the last step is usually division—dividing by the coefficient of the variable term. It could also be multiplication by the reciprocal, if the coefficient is a fraction. If the coefficient of the variable term is 1, then no division is necessary. To succeed at this TEAS task, you'll need to practice solving a range of equations with one variable.

Algebraic equations with one variable can have one or more terms in that same variable. For example:

$x + 2 = 5$

$3x - 6 = -5x + 8$

The x, $3x$, and $-5x$ are variable terms. Constants also are included in an equation with one variable. In the examples given, the constants are 2, 5, –6, and 8.

To solve equations with one variable, you must get all variable terms on one side of the equation and all constants on the other side. Which side doesn't matter; just make sure variables and constants end up on opposite sides of the equals sign. This is accomplished by using *inverse operations* to "undo," or move, variable or constant terms.

Inverse mathematical operations are the opposites of each other. Addition undoes subtraction, and vice versa; division undoes multiplication, and vice versa. One somewhat unusual inverse operation is when the coefficient of a variable on the last step is a fraction. It is okay to divide by the fraction, but dividing by a fraction also can be done by multiplying by the fraction's reciprocal.

The following examples illustrate using inverse operations to solve algebraic equations with one variable.

Solve: x + 20 = 100

$x + 20 = 100$	Subtract 20 from both sides to get the constants **20** and **100** on the opposite side of the = from the **x**. Subtraction "undoes" the **+20**.
$x + 20 - 20 = 100 - 20$	
$x = 80$	Check your work: $80 + 20 = 100$

Solve: x – 5 = -12

$x - 5 = -12$	Add 5 to both sides to get the constants **-5** and **-12** on the opposite side of the variable term *x*. Addition "undoes" the **-5**.
$x - 5 + 5 = -12 + 5$	
$x = -7$	Check your work: $-7 - 5 = -12$

This objective includes, but is not limited to, the following examples of knowledge, skills, and abilities.

- *Understand the meaning of a variable.*
- *Understand the structure of an algebraic equation.*
- *Demonstrate knowledge of inverse arithmetic operations.*

Key terms

algebraic equation. A mathematic equation that includes one or more variables.

combine like terms. Simplifying an expression by using the distributive property.

constant. A number that is not "attached to," or does not multiply, a variable.

inverse arithmetic operations. Mathematic operations that undo each other.

reciprocal. One divided by the original number, or, for a nonzero fraction a/b, the reciprocal is b/a.

variable. A letter, often x, y, or z, that stands for an unspecified quantity.

variable terms. Numeric values consisting of variables and coefficients or constants.

Solve: 5x = 2

$5x = 2$ $\frac{5}{5}x = \frac{2}{5}$	Divide both sides by 5. This undoes the multiplication between the **5** and the **x** in **5x**.
$x = \frac{2}{5}$	Check your work: $\frac{5}{1} \times \frac{2}{5} = \frac{10}{5} = 2$

Solve: $\frac{2}{7}x = 4$

$\frac{2}{7}x = 4$	Multiply both sides by $\frac{7}{2}$ because $\frac{7}{2} \times \frac{2}{7} = 1$, and $1 \times x = x$, so this gets x by itself on the left side of the equation.
$\frac{7}{2} \times \frac{2}{7}x = 4 \times \frac{7}{2}$	The right side can be simplified by multiplying $\frac{4}{1} \times \frac{7}{2}$, which equals 14.
$x = 14$	Check your work: $\frac{2}{7} \times \frac{14}{1} = \frac{28}{7} = 4$

Solve: 3x + 5 = 2x + 1

$3x + 5 = 2x + 1$	Subtract $2x$ from both sides to get the variable terms on the left side of the equation. Subtract 5 from both sides to get the constants on opposite side of the equation as the variable terms.
$3x - 2x + 5 = 2x - 2x + 1$	
$x + 5 = 1$	
$x + 5 - 5 = 1 - 5$	
$x = -4$	Check your work: $(3 \times -4) + 5 = (2 \times -4) + 1$ $-12 + 5 = -8 + 1$ $-7 = -7$

M.1.4 Practice problems

1. $x - 5 = 32$

   Solve the equation above. Which of the following is correct?

   A. 22
   B. 37
   C. 27
   D. 42

2. Solve: $x + 7 = -3x$
3. Solve: $3x = 10$
4. Solve: $\frac{8}{5}x = 6$

5. Given the equation $2x - 3 = 5x + 4$, which of the following is an acceptable first step toward solving the equation?

   A. Subtract 3 from both sides of the equation.
   B. Add 4 to both sides of the equation.
   C. Subtract $2x$ from both sides of the equation.
   D. Add $5x$ to both sides of the equation.

M.1.5 *Solve real world one- or multi-step problems with rational numbers.*

Mathematics is a tool we use to observe the world around us, collect and analyze data about our world, and help answer questions and solve problems. Many simple problems can be solved with one or two steps using simple rational numbers. Being able to recognize the patterns used in these problems will make the solutions easier. Repeated practice will help this process to become automatic and prepare you for success at this TEAS task.

Most problems you encounter will not include specific instructions to guide you to a solution. Careful reading of the prompt is necessary to determine what the question is, what information is relevant, and what details are extraneous. Many word problems will attempt to mirror real-life, professional situations. You must have the background knowledge relevant to the context, choose the correct mathematical operations, and choose a correct sequence of steps, including checking the reasonableness of your solution.

Think about a story told to you by several of your friends. It will include much more than just a few simple subjects and verbs. The sentences contain details that make the story interesting but are not strictly necessary to tell you what happened. These are the extraneous details. The stories might contain conflicting accounts of what happened due to having multiple observers. These could be erroneous details. It is up to you, the listener, to pick out what is necessary in order to understand and remember the story. The same thing happens when you read a math problem, typically called "word" or "story" problems.

It's a good idea to begin a list of verbs and nouns that are generally associated with specific mathematic operations. Think of words like "sum" (+), "difference" (-), "product" (×), and "quotient" (/). Now what do these make you think of for math operations: half, triple, less, more, increase, decrease, total, reduce, factor, and substitute? As you go through this review, try keeping a list of all the words that tell you what operation to use.

Rational numbers are used in these problems. Rational numbers can be represented by fractions. This includes whole numbers, positives and negatives, zero, and all decimals that either terminate or repeat. Irrational numbers, such as the square root of five, will not concern us at this point.

Most problems you are asked to solve will be in a real-world context. In the real world, you will likely not have a boss that says, "Solve these 10 quadratic equations and have them on my desk by 5 o'clock." Instead, you will have to take information from several sources, analyze it, determine what the question is that you need to solve, pick out the pertinent information, choose the correct procedure, solve the problem mathematically, and check the reasonableness of the answer. This takes practice

This objective includes, but is not limited to, the following examples of knowledge, skills, and abilities.

- *Differentiate among necessary, erroneous, and extraneous information in a word problem.*
- *Determine the necessary operation(s) from contextual clues in a word problem.*
- *Perform arithmetic operations with rational numbers in a real-world context.*
- *Check the reasonableness of the solution to a problem.*
- *Solve equations in one variable in a real-world context.*

Key terms

contextual. Related to surrounding content.

erroneous. Incorrect.

extraneous. Irrelevant.

operation. A mathematical action.

repeat. Do again.

solution. The answer.

terminate. To end.

M.1.5 Practice problems

1. George wants to use square pavers that are 6 inches on each side to completely surround his flower garden. The garden is 12 feet long and 3 feet wide. How many pavers should George buy?

2. A cat owner gets a vitamin prescription from his veterinarian that lists the dosage as 5 mL twice a day. The bottle contains 300 cc. How many days will the bottle last?

M.1.6 *Solve real-world problems involving percentages.*

This objective includes, but is not limited to, the following examples of knowledge, skills, and abilities.

- *Define percent in terms of a real-world context.*
- *Calculate the percent of a number in terms of a real-world context.*
- *Find percent of increase or decrease between two numbers in terms of a real-world context.*

Key terms

percent decrease. The negative difference between two numbers, divided by the first number, multiplied by 100.

percent increase. The positive difference between two numbers, divided by the first number, multiplied by 100.

Percentage is a form of number quantity. For this task on the TEAS, you'll need to understand what percentage means in real-world contexts, as well as how to work with percentages within these contexts. You will have to find percentage of a number quantity, as well as percent increase or decrease. Utilize the problem-solving skills discussed in the previous chapter and, if needed, search the Internet for additional practice problems of these types.

Percent means "per 100," or a value's proportional equivalent compared to 100. One percent can be interpreted as one one-hundredth of something. Examples of percent expressions are 45%, 23.8%, 100%, and 0.05%.

When a percent is less than or equal to 100%, then you can say "out of" 100. For example, 50% is 50 out of 100. But if a percent is more than 100%, you need to rethink the wording. It doesn't make sense to say that 150% is 150 out of 100. 150% is 150 for each 100. For example, 150% of 10 is 15.

Below are 100 small squares, and 50 have been shaded.

One way to describe the shading it to say 50% has been shaded—in other words, 50 out of 100. Likewise, 50 cents is 50% of 100 cents (or 50% of $1.00).

Other real-word percentage contexts include: percent off for a sale price; annual percent interest rates at a bank; annual percent gain or loss for a company or business; percent commission for a salesperson; percent depreciation of assets; percentages of ingredients in a mixture or recipe.

Another consideration is finding a percent of a number. For instance, you might need to pay sales tax on a purchased item. The cash register and cashier will do it automatically, but you should have at least a rough idea of what it should be. If you buy about $50 worth of groceries and the sales tax rate is 8%, the sales tax in addition to the $50 is $4. To figure a percent of a number, you convert the percent to a decimal, then multiply the percent times the original number. In this case, 8% is 0.08 as a decimal (move the decimal to the left two places in the 8). When you multiply 0.08 times $50, you get $4 for the tax. So your total bill of groceries plus tax will be $54.

Another application is percent increase or decrease. In a sense, sales tax is a percent increase. You are essentially increasing the cost of an item by a certain percentage. The 8% sales tax problem described earlier means a percent increase of 8% on the total cost of the purchase.

An example of a percent decrease is purchasing an item on sale. If an item is on sale for 20% off, the cost of the item (before sales tax) is decreased by 20%. If an item has a regular price of $70 and is on sale at 20% off, you need to find 20% of the price and subtract. Multiply $70 by 0.2 to get $14, then take $70 − $14 to get $56, the reduced price. (Alternatively, you could find 80% of the regular price. So $70 times 0.8 is $56.)

M.1.6 Practice problems

1. Your current salary is $50,000. Next year you will get a 4% increase in your salary. How much more money will you make next year?

2. Which of the following is 25% of 680 pounds?

   A. 1,700 pounds

   B. 510 pounds

   C. 68 pounds

   D. 170 pounds

3. While shopping, you find a shirt that is marked 30% off. If the regular price is $45, which of the following is the reduced price?

   A. $13.50

   B. $15

   C. $31.50

   D. $33.75

M.1.7 *Apply estimation strategies and rounding rules to real-world problems.*

While the U.S. still clings to standard measurements, you will work primarily with the metric system in medical studies. And for the purposes of the estimation strategies and rounding rules described by this TEAS task, you'll be using metric measurements. It can be helpful to practice thinking metrically in your daily life as well, such as when you shop and drive. You'll also want to be practiced at using rounding rules and estimation strategies when solving word problems.

First, you must have knowledge of some simple approximations for common metric units. Study the following table.

Metric unit	A household approximation
Millimeter (mm)	The thickness of a dime
Centimeter (cm)	The width of an average pinkie fingernail
Meter (m)	The average adult is 1.5 to 2 m tall
Kilometer (km)	The average adult walks 1 km in about 15 minutes
Gram (g)	The weight of one aspirin tablet
Kilogram (kg)	A 5-pound bag of sugar weighs just over 2 kg
Degrees Celsius (° C)	Zero is freezing, 10 is not. 20 is warm, and 30 is hot!

Note that metric units do not have a period after them. Volume is measured in cubic units, such as cubic centimeters (cm³). The exponent 3 is used for metric volume, and the abbreviation cu. is usually used for standard system units. Liquid volume is measured in liters (L) or milliliters (mL). Because carbonated beverages are sold in 2-liter bottles, this is one conversion you are probably already familiar with. One liter contains 1,000 milliliters or 1,000 cubic centimeters (1 L = 1,000 mL = 1000 cc). Helpful tip: 1 cc is the same as 1 mL.

Estimating and rounding are two skills that make many problems quicker and easier to solve. Good judgment should be used when deciding if estimating and rounding are appropriate. Sometimes a "ballpark" figure is reasonable. Even in a laboratory setting, where precision and accuracy are extremely important, a quick estimate can tell you whether you have the decimal point in the right place and can help determine if your mathematical procedure was correct. Estimation strategies that you should be familiar with include front-end estimation, in which you focus on the first digits of numbers when adding or subtracting, and solving a simpler problem. There are plenty of good examples of solving a simpler problem and other estimation strategies available on the Internet, so be sure to search these key words and familiarize yourself with these strategies.

This objective includes, but is not limited to, the following examples of knowledge, skills, and abilities.

- *Estimate metric measurements (e.g., area, length, weight, volume).*
- *Know when it is appropriate to use a given estimation or rounding procedure.*
- *Know rounding rules (e.g., rounding to ones, tenths, hundredths; rounding fractions and mixed numbers).*
- *Demonstrate knowledge of estimation strategies (e.g., using a simpler problem).*

Key terms

estimation. A rough calculation of numbers.

metric system. International System of Units (French: Système international d'unités, SI) based on powers of ten.

rounding. Simplifying a number by removing decimal places or changing those places to zero.

The decimal place you need to round to depends on the problem you are working on. When rounding to a decimal place, such as the tenths or the hundredths place, look only at the digit immediately to the right of the place to which you are rounding. For five or larger, round up. Less than five, drop the digits that follow. Study the table below.

Round	To this place	And the answer is
57.369	Ones	57
57.369	Tens	60
57.369	Hundredths	57.37
0.4983	Thousandths	0.498
0.4983	Hundredths	0.50

When rounding fractions to the ones place, if the numerator is greater than or equal to half of the denominator, round up to the next whole number. If the numerator is less than half of the denominator, round down to the next whole number. Study the table below.

Round to the ones place	And the answer is
$\frac{3}{8}$	0
$\frac{5}{8}$	1
$4\frac{2}{7}$	4
$12\frac{19}{20}$	13
$\frac{14}{3} = 4\frac{2}{3}$	5

Rounding decimals and fractions to whole numbers—which are easier to calculate in your head or quickly with scratch paper—will enable you to estimate if your detailed calculations are reasonable. One frequent error is when the digits are correct but the decimal point is placed incorrectly.

M.1.7 Practice problems

1. Which of the following estimates the answer to $\frac{418.6 \times 3.879}{53.7}$?

   A. $\frac{419 \times 4}{54}$

   B. $\frac{400 \times 4}{50}$

   C. $\frac{4 \times 4}{5}$

   D. $\frac{400 \times 3}{50}$

2. Round the numbers in the table to the place indicated.

Number	Round to this place	Your answer	Number	Round to this place	Your answer
47.38	Tenths		$\frac{17}{33}$	Ones	
$\frac{17}{3}$	Ones		57.44445	Tenths	
6.008	Hundredths		293	Tens	
53,642	Thousands		293	Hundreds	
19.796	Hundredths		99.473	Hundredths	
19.796	Tenths		99.473	Tenths	
19.796	Tens		99.473	Hundreds	
$\frac{17}{35}$	Ones				

M.1.8 *Solve real-world problems involving proportions.*

Proportional thinking is a valuable real-world problem-solving approach. Proportions come up in scenarios from map reading to money exchange rates. To succeed on this TEAS task, you'll need to understand not only what a proportion is, but how to set one up, solve it, and identify the rate of change, also known as the constant of proportionality. The practice problems in this chapter will provide some good examples, but you might want to seek out more practice in other sources as well.

A proportion is a ratio in fraction form set equal to another ratio in fraction form. The numerator and denominator of each ratio are "scaled" up or down by the same amount. For instance, if one ratio is $\frac{2}{3}$, a scaled-up ratio might be $\frac{4}{6}$. Similarly, if one ratio is $\frac{5}{8}$, the other might be $\frac{15}{24}$.

One application of proportion is using a map (a type of scale drawing). If the legend on a map reads 1 cm = 50 miles, and you measure 12.6 cm between destinations, a proportion can be used to calculate how many miles (*x*) are represented by 12.6 cm. In this case, $\frac{50 \text{ mi}}{1 \text{ cm}} = \frac{x}{12.6 \text{ cm}}$ is a proportion that describes the situation. Because *x* is in the numerator, simply multiply both sides by 12.6 cm. On the left, cm units divide out, so you're left with $\frac{50 \text{ mi} \times 12.6 \text{ cm}}{1 \text{ cm}} = x$. Simplifying the left side yields *x* = 630 miles.

$$\frac{50 \text{ mi}}{1 \text{ cm}} = \frac{x}{12.6 \text{ cm}} \rightarrow \frac{50 \text{ mi} \times 12.6 \text{ cm}}{1 \text{ cm}} = \frac{x \times \cancel{12.6 \text{ cm}}}{\cancel{12.6 \text{ cm}}} \rightarrow \frac{50 \text{ mi} \times 12.6 \cancel{\text{ cm}}}{1 \cancel{\text{ cm}}} = x \rightarrow 630 \text{ mi} = x$$

Additional characteristics are direct proportion and constant of proportionality. If one variable is always the product of the other and a constant, the two are said to be directly proportional. *x* and *y* are directly proportional if the ratio is constant. An equation can be written as *y* = *k* × *x*, where *k* is the constant of proportionality.

You might also recall from studying linear equations, lines can be in the form of *y* = *mx* + *b* (slope-intercept form). When *b* = 0 (*y*-intercept = 0), the equation becomes *y* = *mx* (i.e., *y* = *k* × *x*). Since *m* is the slope, in the case where *b* = 0, *m* is playing the role of the constant of proportionality *k*.

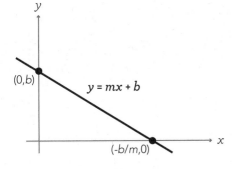

This objective includes, but is not limited to, the following examples of knowledge, skills, and abilities.

- *Define proportion.*
- *Set up a proportion.*
- *Solve a proportion.*
- *Identify a constant of proportionality.*

Key terms

constant of proportionality. The ratio between two quantities.

proportion. An equality of two ratios.

solve. Find the answer.

M.1.8 Practice problems

1. Micah spends 17 hours in a 2-week period practicing piano. At this rate, how many hours will he practice in 5 weeks?

2. The success rate for a salesperson is 1 out of 8 calls. At this rate, how many sales would the salesperson expect to get out of 32 calls?

   A. 8
   B. 256
   C. 0.128
   D. 4

3. A company found an average of 5 defective televisions for every 1,000 checked. If the company produced 85,000 televisions in 1 year, how many of them would be expected to be defective?

   A. 425
   B. 5,000
   C. 85
   D. 0.005

M.1.9 *Solve real-world problems involving ratios and rates of change.*

This objective includes, but is not limited to, the following examples of knowledge, skills, and abilities.

- *Define ratio.*
- *Define rate of change.*
- *Determine rate of change in a given context.*
- *Formulate a ratio in a given context.*
- *Convert a ratio to a unit rate.*

Key terms

rate. A ratio that compares quantities of two unit of measure.

rate of change. A rate that describes how one quantity changes in relation to another.

ratio. A comparison of the sizes of two numbers.

unit rate. A rate which shows how many units of one quantity (in the numerator) correspond to one unit of the second quantity (in the denominator), such as miles/hour.

A popular question in every math class is, "When are we ever going to use this?" Ratios and rates are one part of math that is used on a daily basis. How often do you ask the following?

Question	Answer
"How much does that job pay?"	dollars/hour
"What is the speed limit on this road?"	miles/hour
"Have I had too much coffee?"	cups/day
"Is my cell phone plan adequate?"	gigabytes/month
"Can I afford to attend that college?"	(tuition + room and board)/semester

It is the nature of our world today to think in terms of ratios and rates. Fortunately, the mathematical procedures for working with ratios and rates are quite simple. On the TEAS, you'll encounter a range of real-world problems that involve ratios and rates of change, so you'll want to understand these concepts and how to put them into practice.

A ratio is simply a fraction, which has a numerator and denominator. It might not be in lowest terms. Examples of ratios include $\frac{3}{4}$, $\frac{7}{15}$, and $\frac{11}{9}$. If words or units are attached to the numerator and denominator, then it becomes a rate. Examples of rates include $\frac{5\ days}{2\ weeks}$, $\frac{23\ miles}{1\ gallon}$, and $\frac{3\ teaspoons}{2\ cups}$. Because a rate contains two numbers with units, we can think of these as two variables and imagine them plotted on a graph. The y–coordinate is the numerator and the x–coordinate is the denominator.

Kevin keeps a chart on the miles he has driven back and forth to school since the beginning of the quarter.

By the end of the third week, he had driven 42 miles, and by the end of the seventh week a total of 98 miles. Now let's find the slope of the line between these two points. Remember slope equals the change in the y-coordinates divided by the change in the x-coordinates, or $= \frac{\Delta y}{\Delta x}$. The slope of the line between (3 weeks, 42 miles) and (7 weeks, 98 miles) is found this way:

$$m = \frac{(98 - 42)\ miles}{(7 - 3)\ weeks}$$

$$m = \frac{56\ miles}{4\ weeks}$$

$$m = \frac{14\ miles}{1\ week}$$

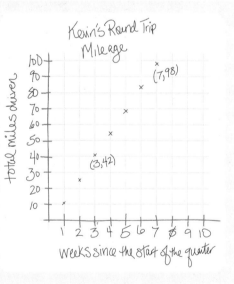

When dealing with rates, we call the slope of the line between two points the *rate of change*. It is not necessary to make the graph to find the rate of change. Just find the slope between the two rates.

> Timmy only likes blue and red candies. In his bag containing 412 candies, he counts 57 red candies and 98 blue candies. We can write several ratios from this information.
>
> Ratio of reds to blues is $\frac{57}{98}$.
>
> Ratio of blues to reds is $\frac{98}{57}$.
>
> Ratio of reds to all candies is $\frac{57}{412}$.

Mike manages a small crew of men at the local utility company. Today they have to go out and cut up some trees that fell on electric lines in a nearby neighborhood. The chainsaws all have 2-cycle engines that require an oil-and-gasoline fuel mixture. Normally, Mike mixes up the fuel in a 5-gallon container in the shop before heading to the job site. He knows the ratio of oil to gas is 1:50. This means that a 5-gallon container should have 12.8 fluid ounces of oil added to the 5 gallons of gasoline. Today is a small job and he plans to only take a 1-gallon container. He calculates the unit rate this way. A unit rate is a fraction with a one in the denominator. Remember that rates always have units, so that means a unit of one in the denominator. The normal rate is $\frac{12.8 \text{ fl. oz.}}{5 \text{ gal.}}$. In order to have a 1 in the denominator, Mike divides both numerator and denominator by 5. This is the same procedure we use to reduce fractions. After dividing by 5, the rate has been reduced to $\frac{2.6 \text{ fl. oz.}}{1 \text{ gal.}}$. This is Mike's unit rate.

MATHEMATICS

M.1.9 Practice problems

Nancy enters a fitness challenge with her friends at work. They all go walking during lunch to stay fit. Nancy decides to track her total steps over 1 month. At the end of the month, she looks back at her records and finds them incomplete. Here is what she sees.

Day	Total steps taken this month at lunch
3	1,248
7	2,912
20	8,320
22	9,152

1. Mary draws several conclusions based on her incomplete records. Which of the following is true?

   A. $\frac{3 \text{ days}}{1,248 \text{ steps}} = \frac{0.002 \text{ days}}{\text{step}}$

   B. The unit rate is $\frac{1,248 \text{ steps}}{3 \text{ days}}$.

   C. The unit rate is $\frac{416 \text{ steps}}{\text{day}}$.

   D. The rate of change is $\frac{416}{1}$.

Carl is thinking of retiring to either Flagstaff or Phoenix, Arizona. He reads in a newspaper that Phoenix has an average of 4,041 hours of sunlight per year out of a possible 4,380 hours (12 daylight hours per day times 365 days per year). Flagstaff has an average of 10 hours and 58 minutes per day. Carl loves the sunshine and wants to retire where he will have the most sunshine every day.

2. Which of the following expressions helps Carl decide where to retire?

   A. 4,041 hours is more than 10 hours, 58 minutes, so pick Phoenix.

   B. $\frac{4,380 \text{ hours}}{4,041 \text{ hours}}$ equals 1.08.

   C. $\frac{4,041 \text{ hours}}{4,380 \text{ hours}}$

   D. $\frac{4,041 \text{ hours}}{365 \text{ days}} = \frac{11.07 \text{ hours}}{\text{day}}$. 11.07 hours equals about 11 hours and 4 minutes per day. Thus Phoenix gets more sunshine than Flagstaff so Carl should choose Phoenix.

3. Find the matching pairs of rates and unit rates.

   A. $\frac{8 \text{ qt}}{2 \text{ gal}}$

   B. $\frac{12 \text{ qt}}{2 \text{ gal}}$

   C. $\frac{10 \text{ miles}}{20 \text{ minutes}}$

   D. $\frac{2 \text{ tsp}}{3 \text{ oz}}$

   E. $\frac{0.2 \text{ oz}}{\text{tsp}}$

   F. $\frac{2 \text{ mL}}{\text{L}}$

   G. $\frac{4 \text{ qt}}{\text{gal}}$

   H. $\frac{120 \text{ miles}}{3 \text{ hours}}$

   I. 30 mph

   J. 40 mph

   K. $\frac{8 \text{ tsp}}{12 \text{ oz}}$

   L. $\frac{6 \text{ qt}}{\text{gal}}$

   M. $\frac{1 \text{ oz}}{5 \text{ tsp}}$

   N. $\frac{84 \text{ mL}}{42 \text{ L}}$

M.1.10 *Translate phrases and sentences into expressions, equations, and inequalities.*

This objective includes, but is not limited to, the following examples of knowledge, skills, and abilities.

- *Define expression.*
- *Define equation.*
- *Define inequality.*
- *Write variables for unknowns.*
- *Determine the necessary operation(s) from contextual clues in a phrase or sentence.*

Key terms

equation. A mathematical statement that indicates the equality of two expressions.

expression. A finite string of mathematical symbols (numbers, operations, variables) that are grouped to show a value.

inequality. A mathematical statement with two expressions that do not have the same value.

simplify. Reducing a fraction or an expression to a simpler form by actions such as cancellation of common factors and regrouping of terms with the same variable.

One of the foundational steps of solving problems is translating written text in the problem into algebraic notation. This involves turning words and phrases into variables, numbers, operations, and a statement about equality. You'll need to understand how those elements combine in expressions and equations. To be successful at this TEAS task, you will need to practice shifting between the concrete and the abstract.

Translating written language into algebra reduces the information to its most basic level. Sentence fragments become expressions, and full sentences become equations or inequalities.

Expressions	Equations	Inequalities
$3x - 5$	$3x - 5 = 70$	$x - 5 > 70$
y	$y = 36$	$y < 36$
$3(2x + 7)$	$3(2x + 7) = 4x - 9$	$3(2x + 7) \leq 4x - 9$

Expressions are made of numbers, variables, and operations. When two or more expressions are combined with a symbol of equality, the algebra sentence is complete.

$5 = 3 + 2$	$12 > 8$	$9 \geq 5 + 3$
$7 \neq 9$	$4 < 6$	$20 \leq 9 + 11$

You will be the author of these translations. Think of this as naming characters in your story, using variables as names to represent quantities.

> Tony goes to a baseball game. During the seventh inning, he buys four hot dogs for $26 for himself and three friends. When he gets back to his seat, his friend Sally wants to know how much one hot dog cost.

This is a story problem. Identify the extraneous or erroneous information. Pick a variable and tell what it represents. This is called defining the variable. Traditionally, x and y are used for variables, but many people like to use a letter that better represents the quantity in the context of the problem.

> H = the price of one hot dog

Decide what the context of the story tells you about the relationship. "... he buys four hot dogs for $26."

> $4H = 26$

> 26 divided by 4 equals 6.5. Tony can say that each hot dog costs $6.50.

Now let's try a more ambitious problem.

"How many dollars do I get for my allowance?" asked the young boy. "Well, if I gave you $12 more than three times your current allowance you'd still have less than $19," says his Dad.

Define the variable.

D = the son's allowance in dollars

Three times the son's allowance.

$3D$ is three times the allowance

If I gave you $12 more.

$3D + 12$ is $12 more than 3 times the allowance

Finally, make the total less than $19.

$3D + 12 < 19$

M.1.10 Practice problems

1. Sue decides to collect postcards. She starts her collection with seven cards. Every week, she buys three more cards to add to her collection. Write an inequality that would allow her to find how many weeks until she has more than 30 cards.

2. Tom is saving money to go to a concert. From his part-time job, he is able to save $18.50 per week. His older brother gave him $25 to start. If W = number of weeks, which of the following expressions represents the number of weeks until Tom has saved at least $235?

   A. $18.50W + 25 = 235$

   B. $(25 + 18.50)W \geq 235$

   C. $18.50W + 25 \geq 235$

   D. $18.50W + 25 < 235$

3. Mary wants to take a taxi to a restaurant. She has only $20 for a taxi ride, plus some change in her purse for the driver's tip. The taxi company charges $2.75 to get in the taxi, plus $1.25 per mile. If M = miles to a restaurant, which of the following expressions represents the maximum distance to a restaurant that Mary can afford?

   A. $1.25M < 20$

   B. $2.75 + 1.25M > 20$

   C. $(2.75 + 1.25)M \leq 20$

   D. $2.75 + 1.25M \leq 20$

Practice problem answers

M.1.1

1. Solutions worked out:
   - 1.22 × 100% = 122%
   - 0.384 × 100% = 38.4%
   - 73.7% ÷ 100% = 0.737
   - 138% ÷ 100% = 1.38
   - $0.516 = \frac{516}{1000}$ where 516 is the numerator and the last decimal place is the thousandths.
   - $1.07 = \frac{107}{100}$ where 107 is the numerator and the last decimal place is the hundredths.
   - 19 ÷ 10 = 1.9.
   - 13 ÷ 50 = 0.26.
2. Option B is correct. This is calculated by dividing 8 by 5, and multiplying by 100%.
3. Option A is correct. This is calculated by converting to a decimal (0.831), then writing the 831 over the place value of the last digit (1).

M.1.2

1. Solutions worked out:
   - First, perform operations in parentheses: 4 + 3 × 3
     Then multiply: 4 + 9
     Finally, add: 13
   - First, perform operations in parentheses: 10 ÷ 5
     Then divide: 2
   - First multiply and divide from left to right.
     30 + 4 ÷ 2 − 2 × 5
     30 + 2 − 2 × 5
     30 + 2 − 10
     Then add and subtract from left to right: 32 − 10 = 22
   - First simplify the numerator and denominator.
     Numerator: 30 − 6 = 24
     Denominator: 18 − 12 = 6
     Lastly, divide numerator by denominator: 24 ÷ 6 = 4
2. Option C is correct. Multiply first: 3 + 12 − 4. Then add: 15 − 4. Then subtract: 11.
3. Option B is correct. Simplify both numerator and denominator first: $\frac{25}{5}$ = 5.

M.1.3

1. If $5\frac{2}{3}$ is converted to a decimal, it becomes ≈ 5.6667. Thus, the increasing order is -5, 0.523, $5\frac{2}{3}$.
2. Option B is correct. $8\frac{2}{3}$ (≈ 8.67) is larger than 8.33.
   - 8.33 is not larger than $8\frac{2}{3}$ (≈ 8.67).
   - 8.33 is not = $8\frac{2}{3}$ (≈ 8.67).
   - $8\frac{2}{3}$ (≈ 8.67) is not smaller than, nor is it = 8.33.
3. Option D is correct. If $2\frac{2}{10}$ is written in decimal form, it equals 2.2. The decimals can be stacked to compare.

M.1.4

1. Option B is correct. To isolate the variable on one side of the equation, you would add 5 to both sides of the equation.
2. Subtract x from both sides of the equation as shown below.
   $x - x + 7 = -3x - x$
   $7 = -4x$
   Next, divide by -4 on both sides of the equation as shown below.
   $-\frac{7}{4} = \frac{-4}{-4}x$
   $-\frac{7}{4} = x$
3. Divide both sides of the equation by 3 as shown below.
   $\frac{3x}{3} = \frac{10}{3}$
   $x = \frac{10}{3}$
4. Divide both sides of the equation by 3 as shown below.

$\frac{8}{5}x = 6$ $\frac{5}{8} \times \frac{8}{5}x = 6 \times \frac{5}{8}$ $x = \frac{15}{4}$	Multiply both sides by $\frac{5}{8}$ because $\frac{5}{8} \times \frac{8}{5} = 1$, and $1 \times x = x$, so this gets x by itself on the left side of the equation. The right side can be simplified by multiplying $\frac{6}{1} \times \frac{5}{8}$, which reduces to $\frac{15}{4}$.

5. Option C is correct. Subtracting $2x$ from both sides gets the variables collected on the right side of the equation. This is an acceptable first step.
   - Subtracting 3 from both sides still leaves constants on each side of the equation.
   - Adding 4 to both sides of the equation still leaves constants on each side of the equation.
   - Adding $5x$ to both sides of the equation still leaves variables on both sides of the equation.

M.1.5

1. Step 1: Read the problem carefully.
   How many pavers should George buy?
   The square pavers are 6 inches on each side. The garden is 12 feet long and 3 feet wide.
   Step 2: Make a drawing of the garden.

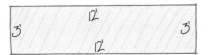

   Because 1 foot equals 12 inches, it takes two 6-inch pavers to equal a length of 1 foot.
   Add six pavers to one of the 3-foot sides in your drawing.

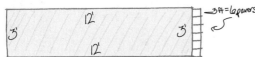

   Next add 24 pavers to one of the 12-foot sides.

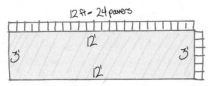

   Notice that one extra paver is needed in each corner to surround completely the garden.

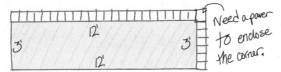

   Step 3: Add up the pavers needed

Length	Number of pavers needed
12 feet	24
3 feet	6
12 feet	24
3 feet	6
4 corners	4
TOTAL	**64**

   Step 4: Visualize walking around the drawing, counting two pavers for each foot. Don't forget to step on each corner.
   64 pavers is a reasonable solution.

2. Step 1: Read the problem carefully.
   How many days will the bottle last?
   The dosage as 5 mL twice a day. The bottle contains 300 cc.
   Step 2: Because 1 cc is equivalent to 1 mL, the cat needs to take 10 cc per day (5 mL twice daily). Divide the bottle's volume by the dosage.
   300 cc divided by 10 cc/day will equal the number of days.
   30 days is a reasonable time period for a prescription. Each day requires 10 cc, and 300 is much more than 10, so you would expect an answer greater than 1. Two days requires 20 cc, 3 days 30 cc, and so on. So 30 days requires 300 cc of the vitamin overall.
   - $\frac{30 \text{ cc}}{10 \text{ cc/day}}$ = (30 cc) × (days/10 cc) = 30 days

M.1.6

1. Convert 4% to decimal form: 0.04. Multiply 0.04 × $50,000 = $2,000, which is your salary increase for next year.
2. Option D is correct. Convert 25% to a decimal (0.25), then multiply 0.25 × 680 = 170.
3. Option C is correct. Find 30% of $45 by multiplying 0.30 × $45 = $13.50. Subtract $45 - $13.50 = $31.50.

M.1.7

1. Option B is correct. Rounding each number to the decimal place of their first digit is a good estimate.
   - Rounding each number to the nearest whole number is a good start, but you are still left with a calculator exercise that is not easy to do quickly in your head.
   - You cannot ignore decimal place value and round to the first digit only.
   - Rounding every number down to its smallest place value introduces more error than necessary.

2.

Number	Round to this place	Check
47.38	Tenths	47.4
$\frac{17}{3}$	Ones	6
6.008	Hundredths	6.01
53,642	Thousands	54,000
19.796	Hundredths	19.80
19.796	Tenths	19.8
19.796	Tens	20
$\frac{17}{35}$	Ones	0
$\frac{17}{33}$	Ones	1
57.44445	Tenths	57.4
293	Tens	290
293	Hundreds	300
99.473	Hundredths	99.47
99.473	Tenths	99.5
99.473	Hundreds	100

M.1.8

1. $\frac{17 \text{ hr}}{2 \text{ wk}} = \frac{x}{5 \text{ wk}}$
   Multiplying both sides by 5 weeks yields $\frac{17 \text{ hr} \times 5 \text{ wk}}{2 \text{ wk}} = x$.
   Simplifying the left side leads to $x = 42.5$ hours.

2. Option D is correct.
   $\frac{1 \text{ sale}}{8 \text{ calls}} = \frac{x}{32 \text{ calls}}$
   Multiplying both sides by 32 calls will give $\frac{1 \text{ sale} \times 32 \text{ calls}}{8 \text{ calls}} = x$.
   Simplifying the left side leads to $x = 4$ sales.

3. Option A is correct.
   $\frac{5 \text{ defective}}{1,000 \text{ TV}} = \frac{x}{85,000 \text{ TV}}$
   Multiply both sides by 85,000 TVs. $\frac{5 \text{ defective} \times 85,000 \text{ TV}}{1,000 \text{ TV}}$
   Simplify the left side: $x = 425$ defective.

M.1.9

1. Option C is correct. The rate has been reduced correctly, and the denominator is one unit.
   - Option A: Mary has written the reciprocal of the unit rate.
   - A unit rate should have 1 day in the denominator.
   - A rate must have units attached.

2. Option D is correct. The only way to compare two rates is to have them both written with the same units. A unit rate is appropriate here.
   - The two rates (4,041 hours per year and 10 hours 58 minutes per day) have different units and cannot be compared.
   - Without units, we do understand what 1.08 represents.
   - In this ratio, the units cancel out, leaving a number without meaning.

3. Correct pairs: A and G, H and J, D and K, B and L, C and I, E and M, F and N.

M.1.10

1. The question asks how many weeks, so let w = number of weeks.
   The total number of cards over time would be $3w$.
   Seven cards to start with would be shown as + 7.
   More than thirty cards would be shown as > 30.
   The inequality is $3w + 7 > 30$.

2. Option C is correct.
   - At least should be greater than or equal to ($\geq$).
   - The $25 is a one-time gift, not every week.
   - Option D gives Tom less than $235.

3. Option D is correct.
   - The taxi charges 2.75 before the taxi starts to move.
   - Option B ensures the fare will be more than $20.
   - The $2.75 is only paid once, not every mile.

M.2.1 *Interpret relevant information from tables, charts, and graphs.*

If a picture is worth a thousand words, just think how much information can be packed into a graph or data table. As the amount of information available in our society multiplies at an incredible rate, a chart, graph, or table can help readers understand the relationship between quantities, how fast they are changing, and the importance of the data. For the TEAS, you'll need to understand the various parts of these graphical displays and how to interpret information from tables, charts, and graphs.

Most graphs you study will be bivariate; in other words, they represent the relationship between two parameters. Traditionally, this is shown as a Cartesian coordinate graph. When plotting a point or reading the coordinates of a point, remember to move from the origin in the horizontal direction first, then in the vertical direction. This ensures a unique point that corresponds to one pair of coordinates. Compare the following graph with the table of points and coordinates.

Point	Coordinates
A	(4,3)
B	(-2,4)
C	(0,0) the origin
D	(-5,0)
E	(-2,-3)
F	(6,-2)
G	(-2,6)

Notice points F and G. Reversing the coordinates results in two completely different points—in this case, they are even in different quadrants.

The graphs you study will not be random collections of points. Graphs tell a story and show the relationship between variables. Consider the graph below.

The title conveys what the graph shows: the number of steps Walter took on Tuesday morning. The x-axis displays the time of day, from 7:00 a.m. until noon. The y-axis shows the total number of steps taken. The scale says to multiply by 1,000, so 8 on the axis represents 8,000 steps. This is often done to save space and make the graph easier to read. Any point on the graph can be read as a pair of coordinates. Can you find the point for 9 a.m. when Walter had taken 2,000 steps? What did Walter do between 10 and 11 a.m.? Apparently he was resting, because the number of steps did not change. Do you see that by 11:30 Walter had taken a total of 5,000 steps? A simple graph can contain a very large amount of information.

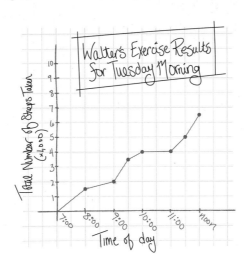

This objective includes, but is not limited to, the following examples of knowledge, skills, and abilities.

- Demonstrate knowledge of the structure of graphical displays.
- Demonstrate knowledge of the structure of data tables.
- Interpret the labels of a graph or chart.
- Interpret the legend of a graph or chart.
- Interpret the scale of the axes of a graph.
- Identify the meaning of a point on a graph in terms of the axes of the graph.

Key terms

axis. A reference line for measurement of coordinates.

bivariate. Containing two variables.

Cartesian coordinate. An ordered pair or ordered triple used to specify a point on a plane or space, respectively.

chart. Information in the form of a table or graph.

graph. A drawing that represents relationships between numbers or data.

legend. An explanation of figures used in a chart.

scale. Ratio of graphical representation to actual size.

table. A set of data displayed in rows and columns.

MATHEMATICS

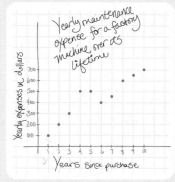

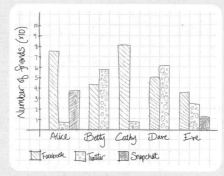

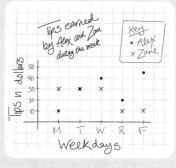

1. Which of the following observations based on this graph is correct?

   A. The cost to maintain the machine is constantly rising.

   B. For the first 3 years, it cost $300 to maintain the machine.

   C. The average rate of change between year 1 and year 4 is $\frac{\$500 - \$100}{4 \text{ years}} = \frac{\$400}{\text{year}}$.

   D. The average rate of change between year 1 and year 4 is $\frac{\$500 - \$100}{(4-1) \text{ years}} = \frac{\$400}{3 \text{ years}} = \$133.33$ per year.

2. Five friends are comparing the number of friends they have on social media sites. Which of the following observations is true?

   A. Alice says, "I'm glad you're all my friends on Snapchat."

   B. Betty says, "There is only one thing missing on this chart: a good title."

   C. Cathy says, "I have the most friends. Look at my Facebook account."

   D. Dave says, "I'm disappointed. I only have 5 friends on Facebook."

3. Use this graph to fill in the two tables and answer the questions.

   Alex's tips

Night	Tips
Monday	
Tuesday	
Wednesday	
Thursday	
Friday	

   Zane's tips

Night	Tips
Monday	
Tuesday	
Wednesday	
Thursday	
Friday	

   On what night did Alex's daily tips decrease from the previous night?

   On what night did Alex and Zane earn the same amount of tips?

   What is the average rate of change for Zane from Monday to Friday?

M.2.2 *Evaluate the information in tables, charts, and graphs using statistics.*

Statistics and data analysis are important parts of what many professionals do quantitatively. Even though uncertainties are involved, these two disciplines help us understand the world of numbers. The TEAS test will require you to understand some basic concepts, and carry out basic statistical calculations. The Internet is a good resource for glossary term definitions, additional explanations, and practice problems.

Measures of central tendency include mean, median, and mode. To calculate a mean, add all the numbers in a list, and divide by how many there are. This is also commonly known as the average, but technically, median and mode are also averages. For example, for 2, 2, 2, 4, 6, 8, 8, 8, you would add 2+2+2+4+6+8+8+8, giving a sum of 40. There are eight numbers, so divide 40 by 8 for a mean of 5.

Median is the middle number of an ordered list. If there are an odd number of terms, there is one middle number. If there is an even number of terms, there are two middle numbers, so the mean of those two numbers is the median. (For the list above, the 4 and 6 are the middle two numbers, and their average is 5. Therefore, the median is 5.)

Mode is the number in a list that occurs the most. In the list above, the numbers 2 and 8 occur equally most frequently. Therefore, 2 and 8 are the modes of the list. This list of numbers is thus known as *bimodal*.

The range of a set of data (numbers) is found by subtracting the minimum value from the maximum value. For the example above, 8 – 2 = 6, so 6 is the range. Range is a measure of spread for a data set. Spread can be determined from a graph as well. The highest y-value is the maximum value, and the lowest y-value is the minimum value. Once these are determined, follow the process above. The spread of a distribution reflects the variability of the data. Observations that cover a wide range have a large spread. Observations that are clustered near a single value have a small spread.

The shape of a data distribution can reveal valuable information, and can be described by the following characteristics.

Symmetry
When graphed, a symmetric distribution can be divided at the center with each half mirroring the other.

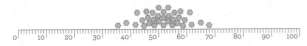

Number of peaks
Distributions can have few or many peaks. A distribution with a single clear peak is called **unimodal**, and a distribution with two clear peaks is **bimodal**. When a symmetric distribution has a single peak at the center, it is referred to as **bell-shaped (or normal)**.

Bimodal

This objective includes, but is not limited to, the following examples of knowledge, skills, and abilities.

- *Calculate measures of central tendency (e.g., mean, median).*
- *Calculate range.*
- *Identify the spread of a data distribution.*
- *Identify the shape of a data distribution.*
- *Identify a trend based on a graph or table of data.*
- *Explain a point on a graph, chart, or table in terms of a given context.*
- *Identify expected and unexpected values (e.g., outliers).*

Key terms

data trend. General tendency of numbers in a set.

expected value. The most likely value of a random variable.

measures of central tendency. Mean is commonly known as the average; median is the middle value; and mode is the number repeated most often.

outlier. A data point that is distinctly separate from other data; unexpected value.

point on a graph. The location of a value expressed as (x,y).

range. The difference between the highest and lowest values in a set.

shape. Symmetry, number of peaks, skewness, and uniformity of data distribution.

spread. The range of values in data distribution.

Bell-shaped, unimodal

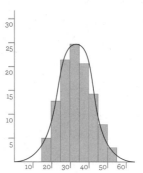

Skewness

When displayed graphically, some distributions have many more observations on one side of the graph compared to the other. Distributions with fewer observations on the right (toward higher values) are **skewed right**; distributions with fewer observations on the left (toward lower values) are **skewed left**.

- **Skewed right**

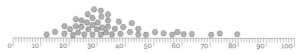

- **Skewed left**

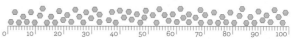

Uniform

When the observations in a data set are spread equally across the range of the distribution, this is a uniform distribution. A uniform distribution has no clear peaks.

Data sets in graph or table form can tell us whether there is a trend in the data. Data trends are usually easy to see in simple data tables, like the one shown here. As the value of x gets closer to 5.0 from either direction, the number of y increases.

Trends are much harder to see in complicated data tables. Graphs are valuable because they make trends easier to see. The graph below shows very clearly that as the value of x increases, the number of y increased, until the value is 5.0. After that, the number of y has a decreasing trend.

An individual point on a graph of a real-world situation has meaning. On the graph above, the maximum point is at (5.0, 90). The meaning of this point is that there are 90 y when the x value is 5.0. Similarly, the first entry can be represented by the point (9.5, 45), indicating an x value 9.5 paired with a y count of 45.

Does value of x affect y?	
Value of x	Number of y
9.5	45
8.0	70
6.5	80
5.0	90
3.5	50
2.0	25

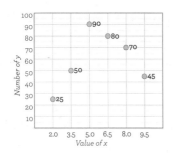

Data set models can reveal what are known as expected values, as well as outliers (unexpected values). The following graph illustrates the outlier phenomenon.

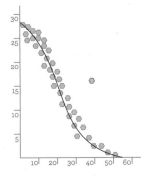

All points on the graph are fairly close to the trend curve except the one that is way above the rest of the data. Visually, we can qualify this point as an outlier, or unexpected value. All of the other data points follow the same trend, and thus are expected values.

M.2.2 Practice problems

1. Find the mean, median, and mode of the following data set: 0, 1, 1, 4, 6, 7, 8, 9, 9

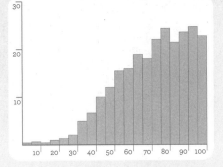

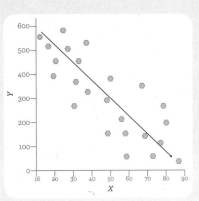

2. Which of the following best describes the distribution portrayed in the graph?

   A. Bell-shaped

   B. Normal

   C. Skewed left

   D. Skewed right

3. Which of the following describes the trend of the data portrayed in the graph?

   A. Decreasing

   B. Increasing

   C. Stable

   D. No trend

M.2.3 *Explain the relationship between two variables.*

This objective includes, but is not limited to, the following examples of knowledge, skills, and abilities.

- *Describe how changes in one quantity affect changes to another quantity.*
- *Demonstrate knowledge that a variable represents a set of potential values.*
- *Identify positive and negative covariation.*
- *Identify dependent and independent variables.*

Key terms

covariance. The way two variables change together.

dependent variable. A variable that depends on at least one other variable.

independent variable. A variable that determines the value of another variable.

The concept of a variable is one of the most powerful ideas in mathematics. Variables allow us to work with quantities that are both known and unknown, from the past, present, and future. A variable represents a quantity that can truly vary. Much of your work will involve the relationship of two variables and how the change in one causes a change in the other. Being able to mathematically describe or interpret this dynamic relationship between two variables is essential for your success on this TEAS task.

Nothing happens in isolation. When you sit down to study for a class, you increase your knowledge and decrease your free time. When you buy a latte, your caffeine consumption goes up and the money in your pocket goes down. When you drive your car, you increase the mileage on the odometer and decrease the fuel in the tank.

Let's use this last example to describe the relationships mathematically. The mileage on your car is a constantly changing number. Every time you drive, the mileage increases. The mileage is a quantity that varies. We can represent it with a variable. Let m = the number of miles showing on your odometer. In between trips to the gas station the number of gallons in the tank is always decreasing. The quantity of gas varies, and we can represent it with a different variable. Let g = the number of gallons in your car's tank. As m increases, g decreases. The variables m and g are negatively (or inversely) related.

> I only listen to the radio when I drive my car. And when I drive, I always listen to the radio. As the mileage on my car increases, my radio listening time also increases.

Again let m = the number of miles on my odometer. Let r = minutes listening to the radio. As m increases, r increases. The variables m and r are positively (or directly) related.

We describe this relationship between variables as *covariance*. If both variables increase, a positive covariance exists, and the variables are directly related. If one increases and the other decreases, there is a negative covariance, and the variables are inversely related.

In all of these problems, one variable depends on another variable. When the first quantity changes, the second quantity changes in response. The increase in the odometer reading causes the decrease in the fuel tank reading. The first quantity is called the *independent variable* and the second quantity is called the *dependent variable*. You can transfer the variables to a graph. The independent variable goes on the x-axis (horizontal axis), and the dependent variable goes on the y-axis (vertical axis).

> As the price of a barrel of oil increases on the world market, the Dow Jones Industrial Average usually decreases. The price of a barrel of oil is the independent variable and the Dow Jones Industrial Average is the dependent variable. This is an example of negative covariance. The two variables are inversely related.

M.2.3 Practice problems

During the 20th century, economists noticed a relationship between the length of women's skirts and the stock market. As the length of skirts became shorter, the stock market tended to go up. And as the hemline fell, so did the stock market. No one means to suggest that one caused the other. Certainly changing fashions are not the cause of the volatility of the stock market. Even though there is not a causal relationship, the parameters follow the same general trend lines.

1. Which of the following sentences best describes this relationship?

   A. The two parameters show positive covariance.

   B. The two variables are constants and represent fixed points in time.

   C. The length of a fashionable skirt is the dependent variable.

   D. The two parameters are inversely related.

The table represents the radius of a circle compared to its area.

Radius	Area
1 inch	3.14 square inches
2 inches	12.56 square inches
3 inches	28.26 square inches
4 inches	50.24 square inches

2. For this relationship, the radius of the circle and the area of the circle are directly related and show positive covariance. Which of the following statements is true based on this relationship?

   A. If these two variables were graphed, the slope of the line between any two points would be negative.

   B. If these two variables were graphed, the radius of the circle would be the dependent variable.

   C. The points on the graph should be connected with a straight line to show that they represent variables.

   D. If these two variables were graphed, the slope of the line between any two points would be positive.

3. Determine whether each statement is true or false.

   A. Every scatter plot is an example of covariance.

   B. The more I study for a test, the higher grade I get. This is an example of positive covariance.

   C. "Practice makes perfect" is an example of direct variation, positive covariance.

   D. "The faster I go, the more behind I get" is an example of direct variation, negative covariance.

M.2.4 *Calculate geometric quantities.*

This objective includes, but is not limited to, the following examples of knowledge, skills, and abilities.

- *Demonstrate knowledge of area as a square measure.*
- *Demonstrate knowledge of circumference as the perimeter around a curved shape.*
- *Understand the concepts of length, area, and surface area.*
- *Calculate area of an irregular shape by finding the sum of the areas of sections.*
- *Calculate linear measures by finding the sum of the lengths of sections.*

Key terms

arc. Part of the circumference of a circle.

area. The amount of space inside a two-dimensional boundary.

circumference. The length around a circle.

irregular shape. A shape in which not all sides and angles are equal.

length. The measure from end to end.

linear units. A unit used to measure length.

perimeter. The distance around a two-dimensional shape.

square units. The area of a square with sides that measure 1 unit.

subtend. Form an angle at a particular point on an arc.

sum. Total of two or more values.

surface area. The total area of a three-dimensional object's surface.

The concepts of length and area are experienced in our daily lives.

How long do the boards need to be for the dog house floor? How much paint do I need to paint the living room? On the TEAS, you need to be able to calculate length and area of shapes (regular and irregular) using various units.

Length (how long something is) is measured with a tool such as a ruler or tape measure. Units of length include inches (in), feet (ft), yards (yd), miles (mi), centimeters (cm), meters (m), and kilometers (km). Both straight and curved shapes possess length. Curved shapes include arcs or entire circles. The length of the distance around a circle (circumference) is calculated by using the formula $C = 2\pi r$ (π is approximately 3.14, and r is the radius of the circle). The length of an arc (part of a circle) can be found by using the formula $C = 2\pi r$, then multiplying by the fraction $\frac{\text{central angle measure}}{360}$ (the fraction of the circle that the arc covers). This is illustrated in the following diagram.

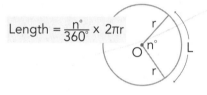

You might need to find the length around a shape, which is known as perimeter. Perimeter is the sum of the individual lengths of the parts of the shape as you go around the shape once. Some shapes have all straight sides (e.g., rectangle, square, trapezoid, triangle). A somewhat more complex version might look like the following.

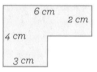

To find the perimeter, simply add the lengths of the sides. To get the missing long side, you would subtract 3 cm from 6 cm, as 6 is the entire span, and 3 is one of the two known parts of the 6. To get the missing short side, likewise subtract 2 cm from 4 cm.

Some shapes are curved, and some have a combination of straight and curved, like the shape below.

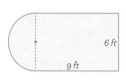

To find the perimeter of this shape, you add 9 + 6 + 9 + the length of the semicircular top.

The length of the semicircle can be calculated by finding half of $C = 2\pi r$, or just πr. The radius is half of 6 ft, so 3 ft. So the semicircle distance is $\pi \cdot 3$, or approximately 9.42 ft.

Thus, the entire perimeter is 9 + 6 + 9 + 9.42 = 33.42 ft.

Area is how much surface space something takes up. Area units include square inches (in^2), square feet (ft^2), square yards (yd^2), square miles (mi^2), and square meters (m^2). Areas can cover a flat surface (such as a box) or curved surface (such as a basketball). Area and surface area have one simple, yet important, difference: area is for 2-dimensional space (flat), and surface area is for 3-dimensional space (curved).

Consider the following table of the most basic area formulas with examples.

Shape		Formula	Example
Square	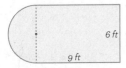 l	$A = l \times l = l^2$	Length = 3 cm $A = 3 \times 3 = 9$ cm^2
Rectangle		$A = l \times w$	Length = 4 in, width = 3 in $A = 4 \times 3 = 12$ in^2
Triangle		$A = \frac{1}{2} \times b \times h$	Base = 5 in, height = 4 in $A = \frac{1}{2} \times 5 \times 4 = 10$ in^2
Parallelogram		$A = h \times b$	Height = 5 cm, base = 7 cm $A = 5 \times 7 = 35$ cm^2
Trapezoid		$A = \frac{1}{2} \times h \times (b_1 + b_2)$	Height = 6 in, base 1 = 6 in, base 2 = 9 in $A = \frac{1}{2} \times 6 \times (9 + 6) = 45$ in^2
Circle		$A = \pi \times r^2$	Radius = 3 in $A = \pi \times 3^2 = 9\pi \approx 28.27$ in^2
Rhombus		$A = \frac{1}{2} \times d_1 \times d_2$	Diagonal 1 = 3 cm, diagonal 2 = 3 cm $A = \frac{1}{2} \times 3 \times 4 = 6$ cm^2

In the earlier example, we can also find the area of the shape using a combination of formulas from the table.

The rectangle area is $l \times w$, or 9 ft × 6 ft, or 54 *ft²*.

For the semicircle, find the area of a circle with a 3 ft radius, then divide by 2. This would be $\frac{\pi \times r^2}{2}$, or $\frac{\pi \times 3^2}{2}$, or approximately 14.14 *ft²*.

Then add the areas, which comes to approximately 68.14 *ft²* for the combined area.

M.2.4 Practice problems

1. Find the area of the shaded region.

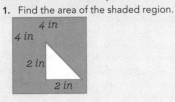

2. Which of the following is the perimeter of the shape below?

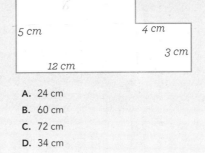

A. 24 cm

B. 60 cm

C. 72 cm

D. 34 cm

M.2.5 *Convert within and between standard and metric systems.*

This objective includes, but is not limited to, the following examples of knowledge, skills, and abilities.

• *Convert between units of measure (e.g., mL and L, fl oz and mL, lb and kg, mcg and mg, mg and g, tsp and L, oz and g, cm and m, Fahrenheit and Celsius).*

Key terms

conversion. Changing one value or unit of measurement to another that is equivalent.

conversion factor. The number used to multiply or divide to convert from one value to another.

unit conversion. Calculating equivalent values between systems of measurement.

In your study and future career, you will deal with numerical quantities every day. Just as important as the numbers are the units attached to the numbers. The importance of measuring quantities accurately with the correct units cannot be overstressed. The health and safety of your clients depend on it. You should be familiar with all of the standard and metric units used in medicine. This primarily involves length, volume, mass, and temperature. The TEAS will test your ability to convert among various values accurately, and you should be familiar with some of the most common conversions.

The metric system was designed to make conversions easier. The units for length, volume, and mass are directly related to each other. The prefixes indicate the degree of quantity of the root, no matter what characteristic is being measured. There are many prefixes for the metric system, but those you will use on a daily basis are limited, and shown below.

Kilo	1,000
Deca	10
Deci	1/10
Centi	1/100
Milli	1/1,000

A kilogram is 1,000 grams, a kilometer is 1,000 meters, and a kiloliter is 1,000 liters. A milligram is $\frac{1}{1000}$ of a gram (a very small quantity indeed). One meter is 1,000 millimeters. There are 100 centimeters in 1 meter. Many students have found it helpful to make a set of flashcards with the same quantity on the front and back, such as 1 meter on the front and 100 centimeters on the back. Just the process of making the cards can help.

To convert between units, use the unit conversion method. Start the mathematical sentence with what you know and end with what you are trying to find. For example, convert 3 pounds to kilograms.

3 pounds	=	x kilograms
What we know		What we are trying to find

Here the needed conversion factor is 1 lb = 0.45 kg. Multiply what you know by the conversion factor (written as a fraction).

$$\frac{3\ lb}{1} \times \frac{0.45\ kg}{1\ lb}$$

The lb in the numerator and the lb in the denominator cancel out, leaving only the desired kg unit in the answer.

$$\frac{3\ \cancel{lb}}{1} \times \frac{0.45\ kg}{1\ \cancel{lb}} = 1.35\ kg$$

Multiplying by a conversion factor is nearly the same as multiplying by 1. This is because the numerator and denominator name the same quantity. Thus, we are not changing the value of what we know, only its representation.

As long as you can find the conversion factor, any conversion can be accomplished. One more example:

Convert 432 grams into ounces. The conversion factor is 1 oz = 28.35 g.

432 g = x oz

$$\frac{432\ g}{1} \times \frac{1\ oz}{28.35\ g} = 15.238\ oz$$

432 g = 15.238 oz

M.2.5 Practice problems

Steve is preparing dinner. He is using a cookbook his aunt sent him from Europe. The recipe calls for 10 mL vanilla extract. Steve only has a teaspoon for measuring. He finds that 1 tsp equals 4.93 mL.

1. Which of the following calculates the needed amount?

   A. $\frac{4.93 \text{ mL}}{\text{tsp}} \times 10 \text{ mL} - 49.3 \text{ tsp}$

   B. $\frac{4.93 \text{ mL}}{10} = 0.493 \text{ tsp}$

   C. $\frac{4.93 \text{ mL}}{1} \times \frac{1 \text{ tbsp}}{14.8 \text{ mL}} = 0.333 \text{ tsp}$

   D. $\frac{10 \text{ mL}}{1} \times \frac{1 \text{ tsp}}{4.93 \text{ mL}} = 2.028 \text{ tsp}$

Jazmine is in Mexico on vacation. While shopping, she sees a pretty scarf in a shop window. The price is marked 225 pesos. Jazmine had seen the same scarf in the U.S. for $18. The conversion rate in the bank window next to the store says 1 peso = $0.06. Jazmine is deciding whether the scarf in the window is a good deal or should she wait till she is back at home.

2. Which of the following describes how to solve this dilemma?

   A. Divide 225 pesos by $0.06.

   B. Divide 225 pesos by 6.

   C. Multiply 225 pesos by $0.06 per peso.

   D. Divide 225 pesos by $18.

3. Match the equivalent quantities below. You can search the Internet for conversion factors.

250 mL	2 kg
88 mL	2.5 cm
4.4 lb	10 in
100° C	88 cc
250 m	212° F
25.4 cm	0.25 L
25 mm	0.44 kg
440 g	0.25 km

Practice problem answers

M.2.1

1. Option D is correct. The average rate of change on a graph is the same as the slope. Find the slope between year 4 ($500) and year 1 ($100).
   - The cost to maintain the machine decreased between years 5 and 6.
   - The graph shows the expense for each year individually. The total cost for the first 3 years is $600.
   - There are only 3 years between year 1 and year 4.
2. Option B is correct. Graphs and charts should have titles so readers quickly know what they represent.
   - Only Alice and Eve have Snapchat accounts.
   - Cathy needs to look at the totals for all sites, not just Facebook, to see who has the most friends.
   - Dave should look at the scale on the y-axis. The scale is by tens. The 5 represents 50 friends.
3. Alex and Zane's tips:

Night	Alex's Tips	Zane's Tips
Monday	$10	$30
Tuesday	$30	$30
Wednesday	$40	$30
Thursday	$20	$10
Friday	$45	$10

   - On Thursday night, they dropped from $40 to $20.
   - On Tuesday night, they both earned $30.
   - The average rate of change is $\frac{\$10 - \$30}{4 \text{ nights}} = \frac{-\$5}{\text{night}}$

M.2.2

1. Solutions:
   - Mean $= \frac{0 + 1 + 1 + 4 + 6 + 7 + 8 + 9 + 9}{9} = \frac{45}{9} = 5$
   - Median $= 6$
   - Mode $= 1, 9$
2. Option C is correct. When most of the data is on the right side of a histogram, it is skewed left.
   - Bell-shaped is symmetric on both sides.
   - Normal is bell-shaped.
3. Option A is correct. As the value of x increases, the value of y decreases.

M.2.3

1. Option A is correct. As the hemline goes up, so does the stock market. As the hemline goes down, so does the market.
   - Variables represent quantities that are changing. They are not constant but instead representative of the entire 20th century.
   - When graphing this, the skirt length would come first and be the independent variable.
   - Because they go in the same direction, they are directly related.
2. Option D is correct. For a direct relationship, as one variable increases so does the other. This would have a positive slope.
   - For any direct relationship, as one variable increases so does the other. This would have a positive slope.
   - The radius determines the area of the circle, so it is the independent variable. When collecting data, you won't always know right away which variable is independent and which is dependent.
   - The relationship is not linear. Because , the area is growing by multiplication and the graph would be curved.
3. Options B and C are correct.
   - Option A: False. If there is no relationship between variables, there is no covariance. If sometimes one goes up while the other goes down and vice versa, there is no covariance.
   - Option B: True, but not because it makes you feel positive. It is positive because as one variable increases, so does the other.
   - Option C: True. The more you practice, the better you perform. At least that's what my piano teacher says.
   - Option D: False. The two variables are inversely (not directly) related. It is a good example of negative covariance. As your speed increases, the results can decrease. Remember this aphorism when you do your math homework.

M.2.4

1. Find the areas of the rectangle and triangle and imagine "cutting out" the area of the triangle. The area of the shaded region is the area left over after the subtraction. Therefore, $(4 \times 4) - (\frac{2 \times 2}{2}) = 16 - 2 = 14 \text{ in}^2$.
2. Option D is correct. The missing horizontal segment is $12 - 4 = 8$ cm. The missing vertical segment is $5 - 3 = 2$ cm. The combined perimeter is $5 + 12 + 3 + 4 + 2 + 8 = 34$ cm.

M.2.5

1. Option D is correct. The answer would be rounded to 2 tsp in the kitchen.
   - The mL units do not factor out to leave tsp. This is not set up correctly.
   - Without units on the 10, it is hard to know if this is set up correctly.
   - This is the wrong conversion factor. Teaspoons are smaller than tablespoons.

2. Option C is correct. $\frac{225 \text{ pesos}}{1} \times \frac{\$0.06}{1 \text{ peso}} = \$13.50$
   - Jazmine did not use the unit conversion method.
   - $\frac{225 \text{ pesos}}{6} = 37.50$ pesos. There was no conversion.
   - To compare prices, they both must be in the same monetary unit.

3. Solution:

250 mL	0.25 L
88 mL	88 cc
4.4 lb.	2 kg
100° C	212° F
250 m	0.25 km
25.4 cm	10 in.
25 mm	2.5 cm
440 g	0.44 kg

1. In which of the following sets of terms are all three values equal?

   A. $\frac{1}{8}$, 0.125, 12.5%

   B. $\frac{1}{3}$, $0.\overline{3}$, $3.33\overline{3}$%

   C. $\frac{12}{5}$, 0.24, 240%

   D. $\frac{7}{1,000}$, 0.700, 0.7%

$\frac{1}{2} + \frac{2}{3} + \frac{3}{4}$

2. Which of the following is the correct way to simplify the expression to a fraction in the lowest terms?

   A. $\frac{1}{2} + \frac{2}{3} + \frac{3}{4} = \frac{6}{9}$

   B. $0.5 + 0.66 + 0.75 = 1.91$

   C. $\frac{1}{2} + \frac{2}{3} + \frac{3}{4} = \frac{6}{24}$

   D. $\frac{6}{12} + \frac{8}{12} + \frac{9}{12} = \frac{23}{12}$

$\left(\frac{3}{4} \times \frac{7}{8}\right) \div \frac{14}{15}$

3. Simplify the expression. Which of the following is the answer as a fraction in lowest terms?

   A. $\frac{4}{5}$

   B. $\frac{21}{32}$

   C. $\frac{45}{64}$

   D. $\frac{49}{80}$

$\frac{7}{9}$, 0.7, -7, -0.65, $-\frac{2}{3}$

4. Which of the following arranges the numbers from least to greatest?

   A. $-\frac{2}{3}$, −0.65, 0.7, $\frac{7}{9}$, −7

   B. −7, $-\frac{2}{3}$, −0.65, 0.7, $\frac{7}{9}$

   C. −7, $-\frac{2}{3}$, −0.65, $\frac{7}{9}$, 0.7

   D. −7, −0.65, $-\frac{2}{3}$, 0.7, $\frac{7}{9}$

$6x + 2x − 3 = 12x + 9$

5. Which of the following is a correct partial solution for the equation and would lead to a correct solution?

   A. $6x + 2x = 8x$
      $8x − 3 = 12x + 9$
      $5x = 21x$

   B. $8x − 3 = 12x + 9$
      $8x − 3 − 9 = 12x + 9$

   C. $6x + 2x − 3 = 12x + 9$
      $12x + 9 = 8x − 3$
      $4x + 9 = −3$
      $4x = 12$

   D. $6x + 2x − 3 = 12x + 9$
      $12x + 9 = 8x − 3$
      $4x + 9 = −3$
      $4x = −12$

6. Mary is learning to use her new exercise tracker wristband and cell phone app. Her stride measures 2 feet, 8 inches. Which of the following is the distance she will walk if she takes 4,500 steps?

   A. 4,500 feet

   B. 12,000 feet

   C. 12,600 feet

   D. 9,360 feet

7. A truck driver is 2 hours into a 1,346-mile drive and has driven 125 miles so far. Which of the following is the number of miles the truck driver still must cover to reach the halfway point of the trip?

   A. 548

   B. 798

   C. 1,221

   D. 1,471

8. A student is shopping for a new Smartie 360 PC laptop. She finds this model on four websites. Site A has the laptop for $612 with 20% off. Site B lists the laptop for $525 minus a markdown of $17. Site C sells the laptop for $570, but the student can save 15% with a promo code. Site D offers the laptop for $500 and advertises, "We never have sales because our prices are always the lowest!" Which website should the student use to buy her Smartie and why?

   A. Site A because 20% off is the largest discount of the three websites.

   B. Site B because $17 is the largest discount.

   C. Site C because $570 − (0.15 × $570) = $484.50.

   D. Site D because this is the lowest regular price.

9. A DJ stores CDs on a 1-foot-long shelf next to her computer. She wonders how long she could listen to her music without repeating any songs if she played them consecutively from beginning to end. Which of the following options gives the best estimate?

   A. One foot would hold about 100 CDs. Each CD is about 1 hour long. Estimate about 100 hours.

   B. One jewel case that holds a CD is about $\frac{1}{4}$ inch thick. One foot of shelf would hold 48 CDs. Estimate about 48 hours.

   C. Three jewel cases take up one inch of space on the shelf so 3 cases/inch × 12 inch = 36 CDs on the shelf. Each CD holds about 80 minutes of music. Estimating 40 CDs times about 80 minutes would be about 3,200 minutes. Estimating 3,000 minutes divided by 60 minutes/hour provides an estimate of about 50 hours.

   D. Measure one CD jewel case. It is 10.2 mm. Converting 1 foot into millimeters gives 304.8 mm. Dividing 304.8 mm by 10.2 mm gives 29.88235 cases. Round this up to 30 cases. The average length of music on the CDs is 76 minutes and 17 seconds. Multiply this by 30 CDs for 2,280.8374 minutes or 38.014 hours.

10. After exercising, a body builder likes to have a protein shake. The label on the can states to use 1.5 oz protein powder with 16 oz of liquid. A full can of protein powder contains 64 oz. Which of the following is the amount of soy milk the body builder needs to use a full can of protein powder?

    A. 0.375 oz
    B. 6 oz
    C. 682.7 oz
    D. 1,024 oz

11. A symphony has 125 musicians. Seventy-five of them are women. Which of the following is the ratio of the men to the total musicians in the symphony?

    A. $\frac{2}{5}$
    B. $\frac{3}{5}$
    C. $\frac{5}{2}$
    D. $\frac{5}{3}$

12. A cell phone user has a plan that charges $0.09 per minute plus a monthly fee of $21.75. He budgets a maximum of $50 for his monthly cell phone bill. Which of the following algebraic sentences represents the limit of minutes for the month?

    A. $0.09M + 21.75 > 50$
    B. $0.09M + 21.75 \leq 50$
    C. $(0.09 + 21.75)M \leq 50$
    D. $50 - 21.75 = 0.09M$

A homeowner keeps track of his monthly heating bill and the average daily temperature for 6 months as shown.

Month	Jan	Feb	Mar	Apr	May	Jun
Temperature	38°	35°	42°	47°	53°	61°
Bill	$71.89	$68.45	$59.34	$54.32	$59.87	$58.93

13. Which of the following conclusions is true based on the table?

    A. $\frac{71.89 + 68.45 + 59.34 + 54.32 + 59.87 + 58.93}{6}$ equals the average rate of change.

    B. The most expensive bill occurred during the coldest month.

    C. The bill for July will be less than $58.

    D. If the homeowner wants to make a scatter plot of his data, he should put temperature on the x-axis and dollars on the y-axis.

14. A basketball coach measures the heights in inches of 10 players on his basketball team. They are 67, 68, 65, 68, 62, 71, 73, 72, 75, and 76. Which of the following statistics about the heights of the players is true based on this list?

    A. The mode is less than the median, and the median is less than the mean.

    B. The median is 68 inches because that number appears more than any other number in the list.

    C. Because there are 10 numbers, there is no median.

    D. The range of heights is 9 inches because 76 − 67 = 9.

15. Which of the following situations shows a negative correlation?

    A. As we move from winter into spring and early summer, the number of daylight hours increases.

    B. A taxi driver watches the miles per gallon (mpg) gauge on her car while she drives. As she drives faster on the expressway, she notices that the gauge indicates a lower mpg.

    C. An office worker notices that the more coffee he drinks in the afternoon, the jumpier he becomes.

    D. A receptionist for a large office in town counts the number of people that come to his desk during each hour of the day.

16. A Norman window is rectangular with a semicircle on top. A classroom has Norman windows in which the rectangle is 5 feet tall and 3 feet wide. The semicircle sits on top of the rectangle. When the window is accidentally broken, the teacher calls a glazier to replace the glass. The glazier charges by the square foot. Which of the following represents how many square feet are in the window?

    A. $\frac{\pi(1.5)^2}{2} + (5 \times 3)$

    B. $\frac{3\pi}{2} + (5 \times 3)$

    C. $\pi(1.5)^2 + (5 \times 3)$

    D. 5×3

17. A basketball player has been recruited from Europe to play for a U.S. college team. The player knows he is 183 cm tall. The college radio station wants that statistic in feet and inches. Knowing that 1 inch equals 2.54 cm, which of the following is the player's height in feet and inches?
    A. 92 inches
    B. 465 inches
    C. 6 feet
    D. 7 feet, 2 inches

18. Which of the following expresses $\frac{3}{4}$ as a decimal and a percent?
    A. 0.75 and 75%
    B. 0.34 and 34%
    C. 1.3 and 133%
    D. 0.075 and 7.5%

$10 + 5(3^2 - 7) \div 2$

19. Simplify the expression. Which of the following is correct?
    A. 24
    B. 10
    C. 15
    D. 7.5

20. Which of the following lists is in order from least to greatest?
    A. $-2, -\frac{2}{3}, \sqrt{2}, 0.5$
    B. $-\frac{2}{3}, -2, \sqrt{2}, 0.5$
    C. $-\frac{2}{3}, -2, \sqrt{2}, 0.5$
    D. $-2, -\frac{2}{3}, 0.5, \sqrt{2}$

$3x + 2 = 5x - 4$

21. Solve the equation. Which of the following is correct?
    A. $x = -\frac{1}{4}$
    B. $x = -3$
    C. $x = 3$
    D. $x = \frac{3}{4}$

$\frac{x}{2} + 5 = 9$

22. Solve the equation. Which of the following is correct?
    A. $x = 4$
    B. $x = 7$
    C. $x = 8$
    D. $x = 28$

23. A student mows and trims lawns to earn money for textbooks. She earns $10 per hour for mowing, and $15 per hour for trimming. She has mowed for 30 hours. Which of the following is the number of hours remaining she must trim to earn a total of $600?
    A. 15
    B. 20
    C. 40
    D. 60

24. There are 28 students in a class, all of whom are taking notes on a lecture. Sixteen students use laptop computers to take notes. Which of the following is the percent of the class using something other than a laptop to take notes? (Round the answer to the nearest tenth of a percent.)
    A. 12.0%
    B. 23.3%
    C. 57.1%
    D. 42.9%

25. A painter is preparing to paint a room and needs to know the area of wall surface in order to buy paint. The floor of the room is 9'10" × 19'8". The height of the room is 10'6". The walls are rectangular. Which of the following is the least estimated area the painter should use to buy enough paint for the room? (Do not figure in windows, doors, or ceiling.)
    A. 860 square feet
    B. 660 square feet
    C. 480 square feet
    D. 330 square feet

26. The distance from Denver to Salt Lake City measures 10 cm on a map. The actual distance is 518.6 miles. If the distance on the map from Denver to Cheyenne is 2 cm, which of the following is the actual distance from Denver to Cheyenne?
    A. 51.86 miles
    B. 2,593 miles
    C. 1,037 miles
    D. 103.7 miles

27. A truck driver averaged 50 miles/hour for 300 miles. If the driver continues at the same average speed for a total of 11 hours, which of the following is the number of additional miles the driver will travel beyond the 300 miles already driven?
    A. 550 miles
    B. 250 miles
    C. 350 miles
    D. 450 miles

28. A mechanic at a bike shop earns $3 for each tire tube repair (x), and $1 for each brake pad replacement (y). Which of the following expressions represents the amount of money the mechanic collects for one tire tube repair and one brake pad replacement?
    A. $3x + 3y$
    B. $3x + y$
    C. $x + 3y$
    D. $x + y$

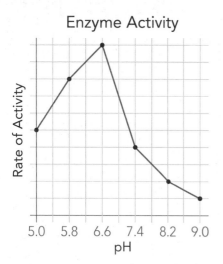

Enzyme Activity

Rate of Activity (vertical axis)

pH: 5.0 5.8 6.6 7.4 8.2 9.0

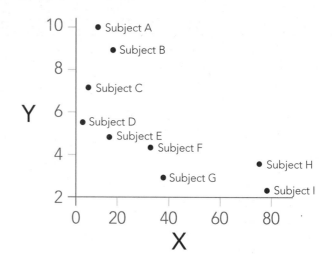

29. Which of the following conclusions is supported by the graph?
    A. The highest the pH gets is 100.
    B. The highest the percent of maximum activity gets is 6.6.
    C. A pH of 6.6 corresponds to the highest percent of maximum activity.
    D. Enzyme activity increases with higher pH levels.

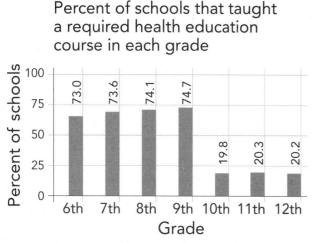

Percent of schools that taught a required health education course in each grade

Percent of schools (vertical axis: 0, 25, 50, 75, 100)

Grade	Value
6th	73.0
7th	73.6
8th	74.1
9th	74.7
10th	19.8
11th	20.3
12th	20.2

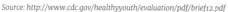

Source: http://www.cdc.gov/healthyyouth/evaluation/pdf/brief12.pdf

30. According to the table, which of the following is the mean percent of schools that taught a required health education course in grades 6 through 9? (Round the answer to the nearest tenth.)
    A. 50.8%
    B. 73.0%
    C. 42.2%
    D. 73.9%

31. The graph illustrates how two variables, x and y, might be related. Which of the following conclusions about the relationship between x and y is supported by this graph?
    A. As x decreases, y also decreases.
    B. There is no relationship between x and y.
    C. There is a negative relationship between x and y.
    D. There is a linear relationship between x and y.

32. A cylindrical well has a diameter of 4 feet and a height of 40 feet. The formula for the volume of a cylinder is $\pi r^2 h$, where r is the radius and h is the height. Which of the following is the volume of the well? (Round the answer to the nearest tenth.)
    A. 251.3 cubic feet
    B. 2009.6 cubic feet
    C. 160 cubic feet
    D. 502.7 cubic feet

Mathematics section quiz rationales

1. Option A is correct. All three numbers are equal. See M.1.1 for related information.

2. Option D is correct. Find a common denominator for 2, 3, and 4. Then write and add equivalent fractions ($\frac{1}{2} = \frac{6}{12}$; $\frac{2}{3} = \frac{8}{12}$; $\frac{3}{4} = \frac{9}{12}$). The answer can be written as an improper fraction. See M.1.2 for related information.

3. Option C is correct. To divide by $\frac{14}{15}$, write the reciprocal and multiply. $\frac{21}{32} \div \frac{14}{15} = \frac{21}{32} \times \frac{15}{14} = \frac{3}{32} \times \frac{15}{2} = \frac{45}{64}$. This answer could also be reached by multiplying by $\frac{14}{15}$ rather than dividing by its reciprocal. See M.1.2 for related information.

4. Option B is correct. By evaluating repeating decimals, positives, and negatives, these are in the correct order. See M.1.3 for related information.

5. Option D is correct. Combine like terms and switch sides. Subtract 8x from both sides. Subtract 9 from both sides. After dividing both sides by 4 in the last step, the solution is $x = -3$. See M.1.4 for related information.

6. Option B is correct. $(2 + \frac{8}{12})$ feet/step × 4,500 steps = 12,000 feet. See M.1.5 for related information.

7. Option A is correct. The halfway point of the trip is 673 miles. 673 – 125 = 548. See M.1.5 for related information.

8. Option C is correct. This is the lowest sales price of the three sites. The final prices of the four options are Site A, $494.10; Site B, $508; Site C, $484.50; and Site D, $500. You can only compare sales prices after the discounts have been taken. See M.1.6 for related information.

9. Option C is correct. This shows good estimating and rounding skills. Thirty-six CDs is close to 40, and it is easy to multiply 40 times 80. Rounding 3,200 to 3,000 makes it easy to divide by 60. Option A is a pure guess. Option B might not be a good estimate of the length of music on a CD. Option D is not estimating. See M.1.7 for related information.

10. Option C is correct. The correct proportion is $\frac{1.5 \text{ oz}}{16 \text{ oz}} = \frac{64 \text{ oz}}{x}$. Cross-multiply and solve for x, which gives 1.5x = 1,024. Divide both sides by 1.5 to get 682.7 (with rounding). See M.1.8 for related information.

11. Option A is correct. If 75 of the musicians are women, then 50 must be men. The ratio of 50 to 125 can be simplified to $\frac{2}{5}$. Option B is the ratio of women to total musicians. Option C is the ratio of total musicians to men. Option D is the ratio of total musicians to women. See M.1.9 for related information.

12. Option B is correct. This equation expresses the terms of the customer's monthly plan – ($0.09 × minute) + 21.75 – as well as the limit (≤) of $50 per month. Option A guarantees that the customer will exceed his $50 budget. Option D finds the number of minutes to exactly equal $50 every month. See M.1.10 for related information.

13. Option D is correct. The independent variable goes on the x-axis and the dependent variable on the y-axis. The bill is based on the temperature. We would not say that the temperature outside depends on Gene's utility bill. See M.2.1 for related information.

14. Option A is correct. The number that appears the most is the mode. The mode is 68. After the numbers are placed in order, the number in the middle is the median. If there is an even number of terms, then average the two numbers in the middle. The median is 69.5. The mean is 69.7. The range should be calculated from the shortest to the tallest. The range is 14 inches. See M.2.2 for related information.

15. Option B is correct. As one variable (speed) increases, the other variable (mpg) decreases. Option A is a positive correlation. As one variable increases, the other variable also increases. Although being jumpy might be considered negative, Option C is also a positive correlation. Option D shows no correlation. See M.2.3 for related information.

16. Option A is correct. The total square feet includes the half circle, which is the area of the circle (πr^2) divided by 2, and the area of the square, which is the length times the width. See M.2.4 for related information.

17. Option C is correct. Cross-multiply the proportion $\frac{2.54 \text{ cm}}{183 \text{ cm}} = \frac{1 \text{ in}}{x}$ to get 2.54x = 183. Divide both sides by 2.54 to get approximately 72 inches, which equals 6 feet. See M.2.5 for related information.

18. Option A is correct because 3 ÷ 4 = 0.75 and 0.75 × 100% = 75%. See M.1.1 for related information.

19. Option C is correct. The order of mathematical operations is parentheses; exponents; multiplication and division from left to right; and addition and subtraction from left to right. Square 3, subtract 7, multiply by 5, divide by 2, and then add 10. See M.1.2 for related information.

20. Option D is correct. $-\frac{2}{3}$ is greater than -2. $\sqrt{2}$ is approximately 1.4, which is greater than 0.5. See M.1.3 for related information.

21. Option C is correct. Subtract 3x from both sides of the equation. Then add 4 to both sides. Lastly, divide by 2 on both sides. See M.1.4 for related information.

22. Option C is correct. First subtract 5 from both sides of the equation. Then multiply both sides by 2. See M.1.4 for related information.

23. Option B is correct. Mowing has earned $10 × 30, or $300 thus far, leaving $300 needed. So $\frac{300}{15}$ = 20 hours of trimming needed. Option C is the number of hours of trimming required to reach the overall total of $600. Option D is the number of hours of mowing required to reach the overall total of $600. See M.1.5 for related information.

24. Option D is correct. If 16 of the 28 are using a laptop, then 12 students are using something else to take notes. To find the percentage, divide 12 by 28: $\frac{12}{28}$ = 0.4285. Convert to a percentage: 0.4285 × 100% = 42.85%. Then 42.85% rounded to the nearest tenth is 42.9%. Option A is the number of students using something other than a laptop, not the percent. Option C is the percentage of students who use a laptop to take notes. See M.1.6 for related information.

25. Option B is correct. This can be estimated by rounding 9'10" up to 10', 19'8" up to 20', and 10'6" up to 11'. Then multiply all the heights and widths of the walls, and add those areas together. Option A includes an estimate of the area of the ceiling. Option D is the amount of paint needed for just two of the walls. See M.1.7 for related information.

26. Option D is correct. Set up a proportion similar to $\frac{518.6}{10} = \frac{x}{2}$ and solve for x. Option A is the scale factor, not the distance from Denver to Cheyenne. See M.1.8 for related information.

27. Option B is correct. Dividing $\frac{300}{50}$ gives 6 hours driven initially, leaving 5 more hours of driving. Multiplying 50 × 5 equals 250 more miles to be traveled. Option A is the total number of miles driven in the 11-hour time period. See M.1.9 for related information.

28. Option B is correct. This models $3 per tube (*x*), and $1 per brake pad (*y*). Option A models $3 for each tube repair, but also $3 for each brake pad replacement. Option C models $1 per tube and $3 per brake pad. Option D models $1 per tube and $1 per brake pad. See M.1.10 for related information.

29. Option C is correct. The point (6, 100) shows the highest percent of maximum activity (100), which occurs at a pH of 6.6. Option A is incorrect because 100 is not on the pH axis. Option B is incorrect because the highest the percent of maximum activity is 100%. Option D is incorrect because the graph increases from pH values 5.0 to 6.6, then decreases thereafter. See M.2.1 for related information.

30. Option D is correct. The mean (average) for grades 6 through 9 can be calculating by adding 73.0, 73.6, 74.1, and 74.7, then dividing by 4. Option A is the mean for grades 6 to 12. Option B is the median for grades 6 to 12. See M.2.2 for related information.

31. Option C is correct. The points on the graph are fairly tight together, following the same curved trend: as *x* increases, *y* decreases. The trend of the points is curved, falling fast at first, then slowing down as *x* reaches higher values. See M.2.3 for related information.

32. Option D is correct. The equation is $3.14159 \times 22 \times 40$. See M.2.4 for related information.

Science

The objectives for the Science section of the TEAS are organized in three categories.

Human anatomy and physiology (S.1)
32 questions

S.1.1. Describe the general anatomy and physiology of a human.
S.1.2. Describe the anatomy and physiology of the respiratory system.
S.1.3. Describe the anatomy and physiology of the cardiovascular system.
S.1.4. Describe the anatomy and physiology of the gastrointestinal system.
S.1.5. Describe the anatomy and physiology of the neuromuscular system.
S.1.6. Describe the anatomy and physiology of the reproductive system.
S.1.7. Describe the anatomy and physiology of the integumentary system.
S.1.8. Describe the anatomy and physiology of the endocrine system.
S.1.9. Describe the anatomy and physiology of the genitourinary system.
S.1.10. Describe the anatomy and physiology of the immune system.
S.1.11. Describe the anatomy and physiology of the skeletal system.

Life and physical sciences (S.2)
8 questions

S.2.1. Describe the basic macromolecules in a biological system.
S.2.2. Compare and contrast chromosomes, genes, and DNA.
S.2.3. Explain Mendel's laws of heredity.
S.2.4. Recognize basic atomic structure.
S.2.5. Explain characteristic properties of substances.
S.2.6. Compare and contrast changes in states of matter.
S.2.7. Describe chemical reactions.

Scientific reasoning (S.3)
7 questions

S.3.1. Identify basic scientific measurements using laboratory tools.
S.3.2. Critique a scientific explanation using logic and evidence.
S.3.3. Explain relationships among events, objects, and processes.
S.3.4. Analyze the design of a scientific investigation.

Remember, there are 47 scored Science items on the TEAS. These are divided as shown above. In addition, there will be six unscored pretest items that can be in any of these categories.

S.1.1 *Describe the general anatomy and physiology of a human.*

This task requires an understanding of the hierarchy of structures and functions within the human body. The lowest hierarchy level is at the organelles within a cell. Organelles perform tasks including obtaining energy from food and reproduction. These roles are central to the cell's survival and function. Cells with the same function are collected into larger groups called tissues. Tissues are collected into organs, which carry out a single task, such as oxygenating blood (lungs) or filtering out wastes (kidneys). Organs work together in organ systems that perform coordinated large-scale functions, such as nourishing the body (digestive system) or protecting the body from attack (immune system). To succeed at this task, you'll need to be familiar with each of these levels, as well as with the terminology associated with precisely locating anatomical structures.

There are many resources available on this subject, including print textbooks, online content and quizzes, and free online textbooks. These are excellent for both learning the concepts and committing them to memory.

Cell parts

Organelles are cell parts that function within a cell. They are analogous to organs in an organism in that they coordinate with other organelles to perform a cell's basic functions, such as energy processing and waste excretion. Examples of organelles are ribosomes, which carry out protein synthesis; the Golgi apparatus, which modifies and packages proteins secreted from a cell; mitochondria, which convert energy present in chemical bonds of food accessible to the cell; and the nucleus, which stores and processes instructions contained in the DNA that tell the cell what its functions are.

Functions of cell parts

Cells with specific functions have varying amounts of specific organelles for performing that function. The specific functions of each organelle combine to perform larger processes for the cell. For example, glands that secrete proteins have a large amount of rough endoplasmic reticulum and Golgi apparatus, whereas muscle cells have large numbers of mitochondria to provide energy for movement.

Cells

Cells are the smallest living unit of life. In humans, some cells function autonomously. One example is phagocytic white blood cells. Other cells work in tandem with similarly specialized cells in structures called tissues to perform specific functions. Examples of tissues are nerve tissues, with bundles of nerve cells specialized to transmit information in the form of electric impulses, and muscles, which work together to move an organism. Cells are highly specialized to perform a specific function, and this is reflected in the relative composition of organelles contained within the cell.

Organs

Organs are structures that are composed of several types of tissues and perform one or more functions. For example, the brain coordinates input from various sources to provide instructions for the body's response to stimuli. The kidney processes blood to remove wastes and to retain electrolytes and water. Bone performs several functions, including providing a framework of support, protecting vital organs, articulating muscle to provide resistance for movement, and serving as a location for the synthesis of blood cells.

This objective includes, but is not limited to, the following examples of knowledge, skills, and abilities.

- *Identify basic cell parts.*
- *Describe the functions of the cell parts (e.g., obtaining and using energy, cell reproduction, cell productivity, cell growth and metabolism).*
- *Know anatomical positions.*
- *Know anatomical planes.*
- *Identify anatomical direction.*

Key terms

anatomical position. Standard positioning of the body as standing; feet together; arms to the side; with head, eyes, and palms of hands forward.

cells. The basic structural unit of an organism from which living things are created.

cellular functions. Processes that include growth, metabolism, replication, protein synthesis, and movement.

directional terminology. Words used to explain relationships of locations of anatomical elements (distal, posterior, medial, etc.).

organ systems. Functional groups of organs that work together within the body: circulatory, integumentary, skeletal, reproductive, digestive, urinary, respiratory, endocrine, lymphatic, muscular, nervous.

organelle. A specialized part of a cell that has a specific function.

organ. A self-contained part of an organism that performs a specific function.

reference planes. Planes dividing the body to describe locations: sagittal, coronal, and transverse.

tissue. A group of cells with similar structure that function together as a unit, but at a lower level than organs.

SCIENCE

Organ systems

Organ systems are functional units composed of several organs. Functions include digestion of food, circulation of nutrients, removal of wastes, and reproduction. The circulatory system consists of the heart and blood vessels. The respiratory system is made up of the lungs, airways, certain muscles, and some of the same blood vessels found in the circulatory system. The two systems coordinate with each other to provide nutrients (food and oxygen) and remove wastes (carbon dioxide). Wastes are also removed by the excretory system, which consists of kidneys, parts of the digestive system, and lungs.

Terminology

Standard terminology to describe the position and location of features in the human body eliminates ambiguity. The anatomical position describes the stance of an individual. For example, an erect human body at rest has the person standing with feet parallel, eyes facing forward, arms to the sides, palms facing forward, and fingers pointing down. Planes of reference divide the body into two portions: coronal or frontal plane indicates front/back division, transverse or cross-sectional plane indicates top/bottom division, and sagittal or median indicates left/right division. Directional terminology is employed to identify the location of features. This includes the terms superior/inferior, anterior/posterior, and lateral/medial. Sometimes two directional terms can be combined, such as posteroinferior.

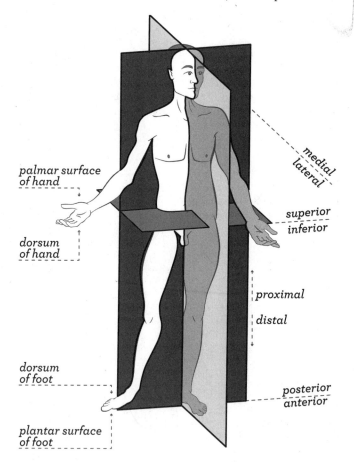

S.1.1 Practice problems

1. Which of the following pairs correctly matches a cellular organelle with its function?

   A. Golgi apparatus – protein synthesis

   B. Smooth endoplasmic reticulum – energy production

   C. Cytoskeleton – movement

   D. Cell membrane – storage

2. Which of the following describes an anatomical relationship between two structures in the human body?

   A. The mouth is anterior to the nose.

   B. The ribs are lateral to the sternum.

   C. The patella is inferior to the tibia.

   D. Muscles are superficial to skin.

3. Which of these organs is directly involved in synthesis of red blood cells in an adult?

   A. Liver

   B. Spleen

   C. Bone marrow

   D. Lymph nodes

S.1.2 *Describe the anatomy and physiology of the respiratory system.*

The respiratory system's main functions are the critical tasks of transporting oxygen from the atmosphere into the body's cells and moving carbon dioxide in the other direction. To that end, the respiratory system is uniquely constructed to maximize surface area for the exchange of gases. (In fact, the surface area of the alveoli in a human lung is equivalent to half the size of a tennis court if stretched out!). For this task, you'll need to know the various parts of the respiratory system and how they contribute to the function of the respiratory system. You'll also want to be familiar with common respiratory problems and how they affect the system's function. Finally, the respiratory system works interdependently with the circulatory system, so you'll need to understand how those two systems affect each other.

The respiratory system mediates the uptake of oxygen for metabolism and the release of carbon dioxide (a waste product) into the atmosphere. The process of aerating the lungs is known as ventilation. Several structures cooperate to form the respiratory system. Air enters through nasal openings or the mouth into the trachea, a large tube reinforced by cartilage rings, which carries it through a system of branching tubes called bronchi and bronchioles (depending on their size) to two lungs located on either side of the heart. Bronchioles terminate in alveoli, which are thin-walled structures that look like clusters of grapes and are the sites of gas exchange. Alveoli are bathed in a layer of aqueous surfactant, which serves as the medium for gas exchange and keeps the lung from collapsing on itself due to surface tension. The heart is located asymmetrically in the chest, marginally over to the left side, which leaves the right lung a little larger than the left. The right lung has three segments, called lobes, and the left lung has two lobes. Each lobe is contained within a tough, protective double membrane called the pleura, with pleural fluid in between. The lungs are therefore described as resident in the pleural cavity. The heart is not a part of the respiratory system.

The lungs are perfused by blood that flows in blood vessels from the heart to bring deoxygenated blood rich in carbon dioxide to the lungs, where oxygen is added and carbon dioxide is removed to return oxygenated blood to the heart for circulation to the rest of the body. Gas exchange in the lungs occurs by diffusion, which is a passive transport mechanism. The rate of diffusion is directly proportional to the surface area involved and the concentration gradient, and is inversely proportional to the distance between the two solutions. Oxygen in the lungs moves into the blood, and carbon dioxide in the blood moves into the lungs. The lungs then exhale the carbon dioxide back to the atmosphere.

Ventilation occurs as a combination of muscle action and negative pressure. The diaphragm and the intercostal muscles of the ribs contract simultaneously to increase the volume of the lungs, decreasing pressure in the lungs. This draws in air. Subsequently, the diaphragm and the intercostal muscles relax, causing a reduction in lung volume and causing air to be pushed out. Periodic inspiration (inhalation of air) and expiration (expulsion of air) from lungs clears out stale, carbon dioxide-rich air, and replaces it with fresh, oxygen-rich air. The amount of air breathed in and out of the lungs is called the tidal volume. A small amount of stale air, called the residual capacity, remains trapped in alveoli after expiration and mixes with the fresh air brought in through inspiration. The breathing control centers of the medulla oblongata of the brainstem control respiration through monitoring carbon dioxide levels and blood pH.

This objective includes, but is not limited to, the following examples of knowledge, skills, and abilities.

- *Identify specific parts of the respiratory system from a list.*
- *Demonstrate knowledge of the function of the respiratory system.*
- *Demonstrate knowledge of the relationship between the respiratory and the circulatory systems.*

Key terms

alveoli. Tiny air sacs in the lungs where exchange of oxygen and carbon dioxide takes place.

asthma. A lung disease characterized by inflamed, narrowed airways and difficulty breathing.

bronchi. The main passageways directly attached to the lungs.

bronchioles. Small passages in the lungs that connect bronchi to alveoli.

cystic fibrosis. A genetic disorder that affects the lungs and other organs, characterized by difficulty breathing, coughing up sputum, and lung infections.

perfusion. The passage of fluid to an organ or a tissue.

pleura. A membrane around the lungs and inside the chest cavity.

surfactant. A fluid secreted by alveoli and found in the lungs.

tidal volume. The amount of air breathed in a normal inhalation or exhalation.

trachea. The windpipe, which connects the larynx to the lungs.

ventilation. The movement of air in and out of the body via inhalation and exhalation.

SCIENCE

Many environmental conditions, genetic factors, and pathogens affect lung function. For example, high altitude depresses lung function due to the lower oxygen levels present. Therefore, people who live at high altitudes evolve over generations to have larger lungs to compensate. Be aware of the effect of environmental pollutants such as chemicals, pollen, and smoke, which can impede lung function through damage to cilia, or cause emphysema, allergies, and inflammation. Genetic conditions such as lung surfactant insufficiency, asthma, and cystic fibrosis can seriously impede lung action. There are also several pathogens that affect lung function and cause diseases such as influenza, tuberculosis, and pneumonia.

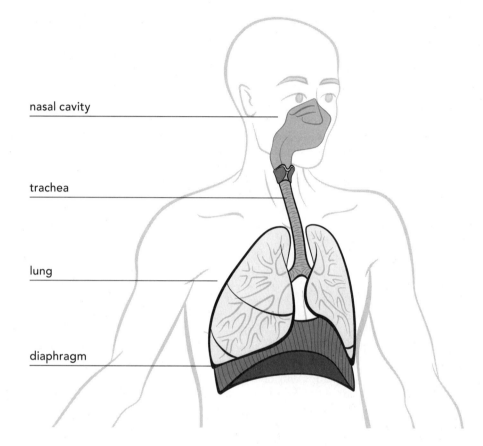

S.1.2 Practice problems

1. At the end of a sprint, a runner breathes hard because the medulla oblongata senses which of the following?

   A. Low oxygen levels in blood

   B. Low carbon dioxide levels in blood

   C. Blood becoming more alkaline

   D. Blood becoming more acidic.

2. Which of the following situations would result in increased oxygen diffusion from alveoli into blood?

   A. Increase in perfusion and decrease in ventilation

   B. Increase in oxygen concentration of blood

   C. Reduction in alveolar surface area

   D. Reduction in residual volume of the lung

3. Match the following respiratory system effects to their most probable cause.

   A. Walking pneumonia
   B. Cystic fibrosis
   C. Influenza
   D. Tuberculosis
   E. Mycosis

   1. Coronavirus
   2. Mycobacterium
   3. Gene mutation
   4. Fungus
   5. Mycoplasma infection

Describe the anatomy and physiology of the cardiovascular system.

The cardiovascular, or circulatory, system describes the movement of blood and lymph around the body, which permits nutrient distribution, waste removal, communication, and protection. The circulatory system comprises the closed system of blood pumped around the body by the heart through a network of arteries, veins, and capillaries, as well as the open lymphatic system, which comprises lymph that bathes the interstitial spaces between cells and is circulated through lymph vessels. To be successful at this task, it is important to know not only the structure of these two systems, but also the functions of the components of each system.

The cardiovascular system performs the vital functions of transporting nutrients, wastes, chemical messengers, and immune molecules. There are two well integrated circulatory systems. The closed circulatory system is a double-loop system consisting of thick-walled arteries that transport blood away from the heart, thinner-walled veins that transport blood to the heart, and capillaries made of a single layer of endothelium that form a network that connect arteries to veins in tissues. The open lymphatic system circulates and filters interstitial fluid between cells and eventually drains into the circulatory system.

The closed, double-loop system transports blood. The pulmonary loop carries deoxygenated blood from the right ventricle to the lungs and returns oxygenated blood to the left atrium. The systemic loop carries oxygenated blood from the left ventricle to the body, returning deoxygenated blood to the right atrium. Familiarize yourself with the names of the major arteries and veins and the structure of the heart and its specialized cardiac muscle cells. The heart undergoes two cycles of contractions: systole and diastole. Systole indicates contraction of heart muscles, and diastole is relaxation of heart muscle. In a simplified overview of the heart cycle, the ventricles contract (ventricular systole), causing the atrioventricular valves (including the mitral and tricuspid valves) to close, making a "lub" sound. Subsequently, the empty ventricles are filled by blood pushed out during atrial systole. At the same time, the semilunar valves in the aorta and pulmonary arteries close, preventing blood from falling back into the ventricles, making a "dub" sound, and completing the "lub-dub" sound of the heart. These contractions are controlled by a "pacemaker" called the sinoatrial node, which sends out electrical signals. Arteries have thick walls to withstand the pressure of blood pumped by the heart, whereas veins have walls with a thinner muscle layer and larger lumen.

Blood plasma contains nutrients, hormones, antibodies, and other immune proteins. Red blood cells contain hemoglobin and transport oxygen from the lungs to the rest of the body. Carbon dioxide dissolves in plasma and is removed by the lungs. White blood cells are divided into two main lineages: leukocytes and lymphocytes. You should have an idea of the functions of these major groups of white blood cells.

This objective includes, but is not limited to, the following examples of knowledge, skills, and abilities.

- *Identify specific parts of the cardiovascular system.*
- *Demonstrate knowledge of the function of the cardiovascular system.*
- *Trace the blood flow through the cardiovascular system.*

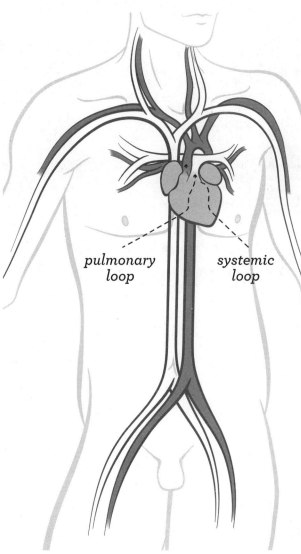

pulmonary loop   *systemic loop*

SCIENCE

The open circulatory system's capillaries drain interstitial fluid that fills the spaces between the cells and filter it through a system of lymph nodes that are enriched in lymphocytes and provide surveillance by the immune system. Lymph eventually drains into the large veins leading back to the heart. Lymph is essentially plasma with the red blood cells removed. Large numbers of leukocytes and lymphocytes are enriched in lymph nodes, where they monitor and respond to foreign molecules washed into the system. Typically, lymph nodes are enriched in oral, nasal, and genital regions where foreign entities enter the body.

You should have a general understanding of pathologies of the circulatory system, such as heart attacks, stroke, aneurysms, atherosclerosis, arrhythmias, and hypertension.

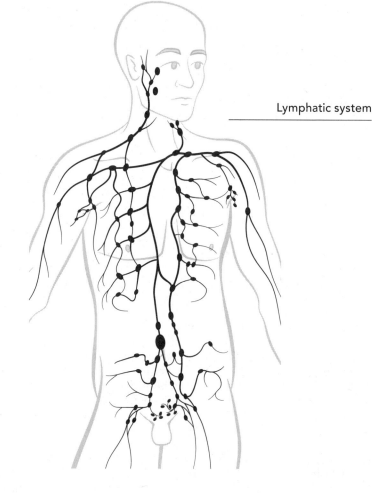

Lymphatic system

Key terms

arteries. Blood vessels that deliver blood from the heart to other parts of the body.

capillary. Small blood vessels that connect arterioles to venules.

diastole. The portion of the cardiac cycle in which the heart refills with blood.

heart. The muscle that pumps blood throughout the body.

hemoglobin. The protein in red blood cells that carries oxygen from the lungs to the rest of the body.

leukocyte. White blood cells, which protect the body against disease.

lymph. Clear fluid that moves throughout the lymphatic system to fight disease.

lymphocyte. A subtype of white blood cell found in lymph.

plasma. The pale yellow component of blood that carries red blood cells, white blood cells, and platelets throughout the body.

systole. The portion of the cardiac cycle in which the heart expels blood.

vein. Blood vessels that carry blood to the heart.

S.1.3 Practice problems

1. Which of the following describes a property of cardiac cells?

   A. Generation of electrical impulses

   B. Production of red blood cells

   C. Immune protection functions

   D. Removal of waste products from the body

2. Which of the following blood component levels would be expected to increase following vaccination?

   A. Red blood cells

   B. Antibodies

   C. Dissolved gases

   D. Leukocytes

3. Which of the following statements regarding the circulatory system is correct?

   A. The sinoatrial node is present in the top section of the right atrium.

   B. All veins carry deoxygenated blood back to the heart.

   C. The heart's "lub-dub" sound is caused by electrical impulse generation.

   D. The heart's atria have thicker walls than the ventricles.

S.1.4 *Describe the anatomy and physiology of the gastrointestinal system.*

The gastrointestinal system is also referred to as the digestive system or the alimentary canal. It is located in the abdominal cavity and is specialized for breaking down food for absorption and distribution to the rest of the body. Specialized regions and glands perform both mechanical and chemical (enzymatic) digestion. Blood vessels absorb the digested nutrients, and smooth muscle is under parasympathetic nervous system control. For this task, you need to know the structure and function of the organs of the digestive system, as well as the enzymes and hormones that control digestion.

Textbooks and online materials are excellent resources to use. You might want to make flashcards to memorize structure/function relationships.

The gastrointestinal system starts at the mouth and ends at the anus. Appreciating regional specialization is the key to understanding the structure and function of the gastrointestinal system. After food is ingested, mechanical digestion by chewing and grinding in the mouth increases surface area by breaking it down to smaller pieces. Mucus in saliva lubricates the food. Saliva also provides amylase and lipase to initiate chemical digestion of starch and lipids. Food then is packaged into small parcels called "bolus" and swallowed (deglutition). As it passes through the pharynx, the epiglottis closes the tracheal opening, and the food passes into the esophagus. Peristalsis moves the bolus down to the stomach through the gastric sphincter, which prevents reflux of food back into the esophagus.

Chemical digestion of proteins is initiated in the stomach by the action of the enzyme pepsin, which is activated by acid and autocatalysis. There are three main secretions of the stomach: pepsinogen (chief cells), mucus (goblet cells), and hydrochloric acid (parietal cells). Following digestion in the stomach, the contents (now called chyme) pass through the pyloric sphincter into the duodenum, which is the first part of the small intestine.

In the duodenum, chyme is neutralized by bicarbonate in pancreatic secretions. The duodenum receives alkaline bile juices from the gall bladder, which helps neutralize acid chyme. In addition, the duodenum produces a large number "brush border" enzymes, including proteases, lactase and other disaccharidases, and bicarbonate. Villi and microvilli in the small intestine (largely the ileum) absorb polar digested nutrients into blood, lipids into lacteals as chylomicrons, and vitamin B12. From the small intestine, blood carrying nutrients passes to the liver through the hepatic portal duct, allowing liver enzymes to deaminate amino acids, convert ammonia to urea, metabolize consumed toxins, and store glucose as glycogen.

The digested material then passes into the cecum and into the large intestine or colon. The vermiform appendix projects from the cecum, which is located at the junction of the small and large intestines. A lot of water and nutrients are absorbed in the small intestine, and the large intestine absorbs remaining water and salt from digested food. The waste from the small intestine is exposed to bacterial fermentation in the colon. Vitamin K is absorbed in the large intestine. The waste accumulates in the rectum and is ejected through the anus.

This objective includes, but is not limited to, the following examples of knowledge, skills, and abilities.

- *Identify specific parts of the gastrointestinal system.*
- *Demonstrate knowledge of the function of the gastrointestinal system.*
- *Describe the role of enzymes in the gastrointestinal system.*

SCIENCE

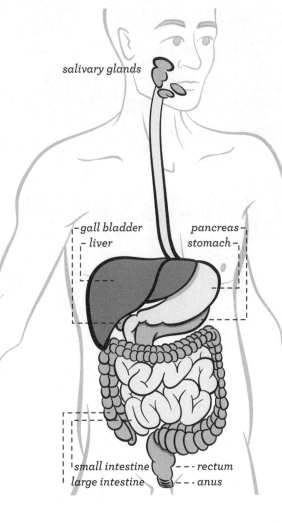

salivary glands

gall bladder
liver

pancreas
stomach

small intestine
large intestine

rectum
anus

Key terms

anus. The opening of the rectum from which solid waste is expelled.

bolus. A mass of food that has been chewed and swallowed.

chyme. The semifluid mass of partly digested food that moves from the stomach to the small intestine.

enzymatic digestion. The break down of food by enzymes for absorption.

gall bladder. The organ that stores bile.

large intestine. Also known as the colon, where vitamins and water are absorbed before feces is stored prior to elimination.

liver. The organ that produces bile, regulates glycogen storage, and performs other bodily functions.

mouth. The oral cavity at the entry to the alimentary canal.

pancreas. The gland of the digestive and endocrine systems that produces insulin and secretes pancreatic juices.

peristalsis. A series of muscle contractions that move food through the digestive tract.

rectum. The last section of the large intestine, ending with the anus.

saliva. The clear liquid found in the mouth, also known as spit.

small intestine. The part of the GI tract between the stomach and large intestine that includes the duodenum, jejunum, and ileum, where digestion and absorption of food occurs.

stomach. The organ between the esophagus and small intestine in which the major portion of digestion occurs.

Hormones regulate many aspects of nutrition. Ghrelin induces hunger, and leptin causes the sensation of satiety. Hormones induce secretions and speed up the movement of food through the small intestine. Insulin induces cellular uptake of glucose, and glucagon stimulates breakdown of stored glycogen. Other hormones and nerve function modulate digestive action.

Resources for studying the complex digestive system include biology textbooks. You should know the general functions and major hormones and enzymes of each organ, but exhaustive detail is not necessary.

Organ	Enzymes	Major hormones
Mouth	Salivary amylase, salivary lipase	None
Stomach	Gastric lipase, pepsin(ogen), HCl	Gastrin, ghrelin
Liver	Bile (stored in gall bladder)	None
Pancreas	Pancreatic juice (bicarbonate, lipase, trypsin(ogen), proteases and amylase)	Secretin, somatostatin, insulin, glucagon
Small Intestine	Brush border enzymes (proteases, lactase, disaccharidases)	Cholecystokinin, somatostatin, secretin, motilin
Large Intestine	None	None

S.1.4 Practice problems

1. Which of the following physiological responses follows eating a large meal?

   A. Pulse rate increases.

   B. Peristalsis rate increases.

   C. Enzyme production decreases.

   D. Parasympathetic nervous activity decreases.

2. Which of the following describes why liver failure is a critical health emergency?

   A. The liver produces the majority of digestive enzymes.

   B. Food is filtered through the liver before digestion takes place.

   C. The liver helps digested food products to be pumped around the body.

   D. The liver filters digestion products and produces urea as waste.

3. Fill in the table below with the names of the structure, hormone, or enzyme that matches the characteristic.

Characteristic	Name
Carbohydrate-digesting enzyme produced by salivary glands	
Zymogen form of protease produced by the stomach	
Cells that produce acid in the stomach	
Valve through which chyme passes from stomach to duodenum	
Hormone produced by stomach that induces stomach secretions	
Hormone that induces bile and pancreatic juice secretion	
Second section of small intestine where majority of absorption occurs	
Blood vessel that carries nutrients directly from small intestine to liver	
Substance mainly absorbed from waste in large intestine	
Region of large intestine in which feces is stored before elimination	

S.1.5 Describe the anatomy and physiology of the neuromuscular system.

The neuromuscular system is a complex system that integrates muscles and nerves. This system affects every part of the body and is vital in controlling involuntary and voluntary movement. This TEAS task will ask questions about the specific parts of the neuromuscular system and how those parts contribute to the function of the system. TEAS also requires you to know the structure of muscles and nerves.

Nerves and muscles comprise the neuromuscular system. Nerves are long bundles of axons that transmit signals from the central nervous system. These signals start as electrical impulses generated at the nerve cell end. The impulse travels along the axon, and then is transmitted to the next cell using chemical neurotransmitters secreted into the synapse from the axon terminals.

This objective includes, but is not limited to, the following examples of knowledge, skills, and abilities.

- *Identify specific parts of the neuromuscular system.*
- *Demonstrate knowledge of the function of the neuromuscular system.*
- *Describe how the nervous system controls the muscles.*

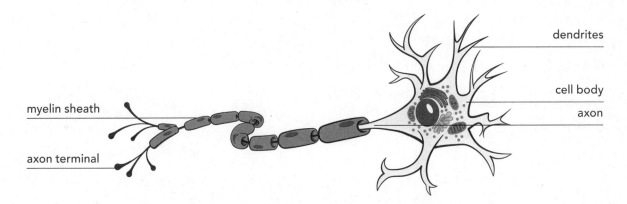

dendrites

cell body

axon

myelin sheath

axon terminal

Nerves send and receive signals in the neuromuscular system. Sensory (afferent) nerves send messages to the central nervous system, and motor (efferent) nerves send messages out to the muscles. The autonomic (involuntary) nervous system controls involuntary actions involving cardiac and smooth muscle, such as heart rhythm, digestion, and breathing. Voluntary nerve signals make skeletal muscles do a deliberate action such as walking, throwing, or typing.

Muscles contain long myofibrils made of sarcomere units, each consisting of long strands of proteins called actin (thin filaments) and myosin (thick filaments).

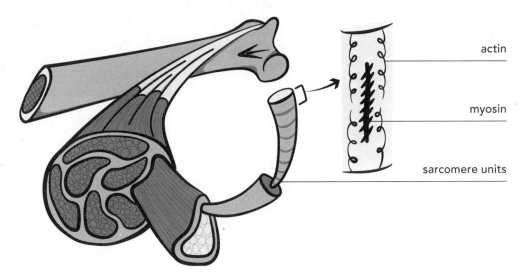

actin

myosin

sarcomere units

Skeletal muscles work by contracting. First, the nervous system sends a signal to a muscle. Actin and myosin proteins in the muscle slide past each other, creating either a contraction or a relaxation of the muscle. These two basic motions are responsible for all muscle movement. Each muscle fiber is connected to a nerve fiber. For the entire muscle to move, it takes a concerted effort by many nerves and fibers and the use of ATP to power the contraction.

Ideally, muscles respond to nerve impulses in very specific ways. Receptors in muscles allow them to receive a signal and respond with the appropriate magnitude and movement. This signal and response can be disrupted by disorders ranging from muscle strain and sprain to muscular dystrophy.

Key terms

autonomic nervous system. The part of the peripheral nervous system that regulates unconscious body functions such as breathing and heart rate.

axon. A nerve fiber that carries a nerve impulse away from the neuron cell body.

contraction. The process leading to shortening and/or development of tension in a muscle.

involuntary. Without intentional control.

muscle. Fibrous tissue that produces force and motion to move the body or produce movement in parts of the body.

nerve. A bundle of nerve fibers that transmits electrical impulses toward and away from the brain and spinal cord.

reflex. An involuntary action to a stimulus.

relaxation. Release of tension in a muscle.

synapse. The structure that allows neurons to pass signals to other neurons, muscles, or glands.

voluntary. With intentional control.

s.1.5 Practice problems

1. Which of the following actions is controlled by the autonomic nervous system?

   A. Walking

   B. Chewing

   C. Heart beating

   D. Talking

2. Which of the following processes best describes how a signal travels across a nerve synapse?

   A. Electrical

   B. Kinetic

   C. Potential

   D. Chemical

3. What is the primary component of muscles?

   A. Fat

   B. Protein

   C. Carbohydrate

   D. Nucleic acid

S.1.6 *Describe the anatomy and physiology of the reproductive system.*

The male and female reproductive systems are complex and involve physical structures, hormones, and secretions. The reproductive system works in tandem with the endocrine system to influence many other parts of the body. The TEAS will ask questions about the male and female systems that require knowledge of the various structures and how they contribute to reproductive functions.

The male reproductive system generates male gametes (sperm) and delivers them to the female reproductive system. Major components of the male system include the penis, vas deferens, urethra, prostate, seminal vesicles, testis (plural: testes), and scrotum. The scrotum houses the testes away from the body to lower their temperature during sperm production. The prostate and seminal vesicles produce the fluids necessary for lubricating and nourishing the sperm. The vas deferens, urethra, and penis form the conduit through which sperm is ejected.

This objective includes, but is not limited to, the following examples of knowledge, skills, and abilities.

- *Identify specific parts of the male and female reproductive systems.*
- *Demonstrate knowledge of the function of the reproductive system.*
- *Demonstrate knowledge of the relationship between the reproductive system and the endocrine system.*

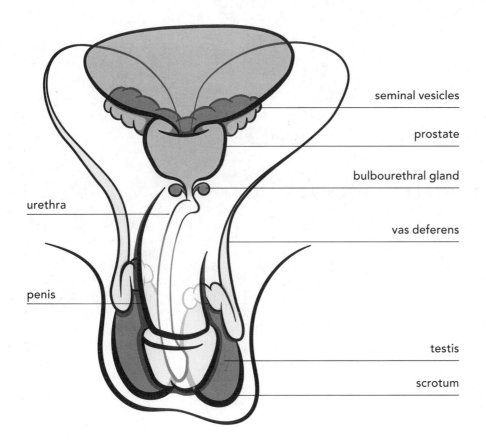

urethra

penis

seminal vesicles

prostate

bulbourethral gland

vas deferens

testis

scrotum

Key terms

cervix. The passage that forms the lower part of the uterus.

estrogen. Female sex hormones.

fallopian tubes. Tubes that carry eggs from the ovaries to the uterus.

ovary. Organ in which eggs are produced for reproduction.

penis. Organ for elimination of urine and sperm from the male body.

prostate. The gland in males that controls the release of urine and secretes a part of semen that enhances motility and fertility of sperm.

scrotum. The pouch of skin that contains the testicles.

testes (testicles). The organs that produce sperm; also called testes.

testosterone. The hormone that stimulates male secondary sexual characteristics.

urethra. The tube that connects the bladder to the exterior of the body.

uterus. The womb.

vagina. The tube that connects the external genitals to the cervix.

vas deferens. The duct in which sperm moves from a testicle to the urethra.

SCIENCE

The female reproductive system generates female gametes (eggs) and incubates the fetus during pregnancy. The majority of the female reproductive system is internal: ovaries, fallopian tubes, uterus, cervix, and vagina. The vagina leads from the external genitals to the cervix, which is the opening to the uterus. The fallopian tubes connect the ovaries to the uterus. In response to changing hormone levels, the Graafian follicle in the ovary matures and releases an egg that then travels down the fallopian tubes to the uterus. Fertilization normally occurs in the fallopian tubes. The fertilized egg embeds itself in the uterine wall (endometrium) and produces placenta that allows the fetus and parent blood supplies to network. The placenta nourishes the fetus and removes wastes.

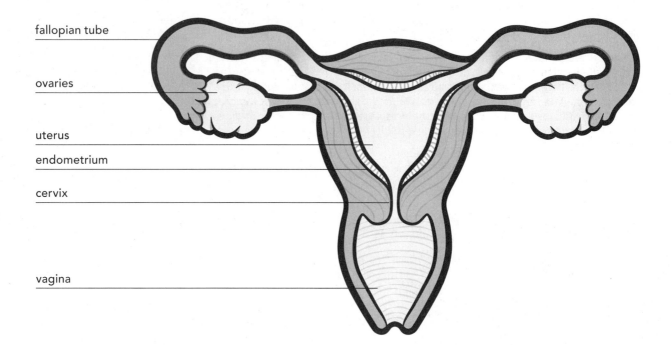

Hormones are part of the endocrine system and allow for cell-to-cell communication. Females produce estrogen from the ovaries, which causes the egg to mature in the ovary's Graafian follicle and the uterine endometrium to thicken. A surge of luteinizing hormone (LH) from the pituitary causes the developing egg to be released. The empty Graafian follicle is now called the corpus luteum and produces large amounts of progesterone to prepare the endometrium for implantation of the fertilized egg. If implantation does not occur, the uterine lining sheds. This cycle of maturation and shedding of endometrium is called the menstrual cycle. Testosterone production is not cyclical, so sperm are constantly produced and matured, unlike eggs. Both male and female hormones help control secondary sexual characteristics, such as production of mammary glands, axial and facial hair, fat deposition patterns, and muscle growth.

s.1.6 Practice problems

1. Which of the following organs produces sperm?

   A. Penis

   B. Testes

   C. Prostate

   D. Vas deferens

2. Which of the following connects the ovaries and uterus?

   A. Vagina

   B. Cervix

   C. Vas deferens

   D. Fallopian tubes

3. In which of the following organs is estrogen primarily made?

   A. Testicles

   B. Uterus

   C. Scrotum

   D. Ovaries

S.1.7 *Describe the anatomy and physiology of the integumentary system.*

The integumentary system contains organs and glands that are vital to protecting the body and regulating temperature. The integumentary system refers to the largest organ: the skin. The TEAS requires knowledge of the parts of the system, its function in excretion, and its function in thermoregulation.

The integumentary system consists of skin, hair, and nails, as well as the sebaceous, sudoriferous, and ceruminous glands. The skin can be further divided into the epidermis (outer layer), dermis (middle layer), and subcutaneous or hypodermis (inner layer). Within the skin, there are hair follicles, sweat glands, and blood vessels. The skin is an important organ in maintaining homeostasis and providing a waterproof barrier between the inside of the body and the external environment. The TEAS will ask questions about the structures of the integumentary system.

This objective includes, but is not limited to, the following examples of knowledge, skills, and abilities.

- *Identify specific parts of the integumentary system.*
- *Demonstrate knowledge of the function of the integumentary system.*
- *Describe the role of the integumentary system in thermoregulation.*

Integumentary system

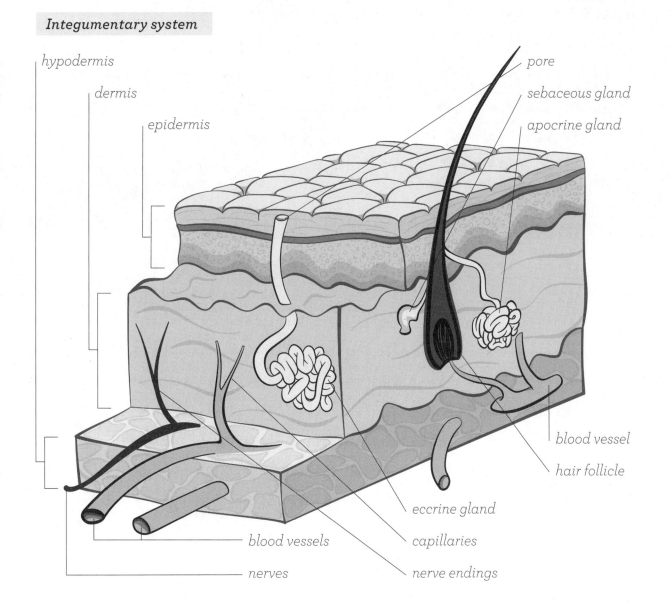

hypodermis

dermis

epidermis

pore

sebaceous gland

apocrine gland

blood vessel

hair follicle

eccrine gland

blood vessels

capillaries

nerves

nerve endings

The integumentary system is responsible for some excretion in the body. Along with water, minerals including sodium, chloride, and magnesium are excreted by the sudoriferous glands. When these minerals build up in the body they are excreted in higher amounts. Sweat can also contain trace amounts of urea, lactic acid, and alcohol.

The skin allows for interaction between the body and the environment. The skin contains sensory nerve endings that allow the body to detect touch, change in temperature, and pain. Skin also produces vitamin D when ultraviolet light hits the skin.

The integumentary system plays a vital role in thermoregulation. When the body becomes too warm, sweat is produced by sebaceous glands. The evaporation of the water on the skin creates a cooling effect on the skin. Blood vessels in the skin can also dilate when the body is warm. The dilated blood vessels carry more blood closer to the skin surface; the blood is cooled and returns to deeper tissue at a cooler temperature. This can look like flushed cheeks. If the body is too cold, blood vessels constrict so that less blood is carried to the skin surface.

Key terms

constrict. To become narrower.

dermis. The middle layer of skin.

dilate. To become wider.

epidermis. The outer layer of the skin.

excretion. Elimination of metabolic waste from the body.

gland. An organ that secretes a substance.

integumentary system. An organ system comprised of skin and its associated organs.

skin. The thin layer of tissue that covers the body.

subcutaneous. Under the dermis.

sweat. Perspiration excreted by sweat glands through the skin.

S.1.7 Practice problems

1. Which of the following is the outermost layer of the skin?

   A. Dermis

   B. Sudoriferous

   C. Sebaceous

   D. Epidermis

2. Which of the following is not excreted through the integumentary system?

   A. Alcohol

   B. Minerals

   C. Blood

   D. Urea

3. Which of the following mechanisms is used when the body becomes too cold?

   A. Blood vessel dilation

   B. Sweating

   C. Blood vessel constriction

   D. Vitamin D production

S.1.8 Describe the anatomy and physiology of the endocrine system.

The endocrine system is a set of organs that secrete hormones directly into the circulatory system. Those hormones regulate many of the patterns in the human body, so understanding the endocrine system aides in understanding the human body. The TEAS will ask questions about parts of the endocrine system, hormones, and the regulatory functions provided by the endocrine system. In particular, you'll need to be familiar with the relationship between the endocrine system and the central nervous system.

The major glands in the endocrine system, from head down, are the pineal, hypothalamus, pituitary, thyroid and parathyroid, thymus, adrenal, pancreas, and ovaries or testes. These glands send hormones (chemical messengers) through the blood to other organs and tissues in the body to control the function of that organ. For example, the pancreas releases insulin, which signals cells to uptake sugar. Without insulin's actions, sugar will not enter cells, causing high blood sugar levels and diabetes. The TEAS will ask questions about endocrine system glands.

This objective includes, but is not limited to, the following examples of knowledge, skills, and abilities.

- *Identify specific parts of the endocrine system.*
- *Demonstrate knowledge of the function of the endocrine system.*
- *Demonstrate knowledge of the relationship between the central nervous system and the endocrine system.*

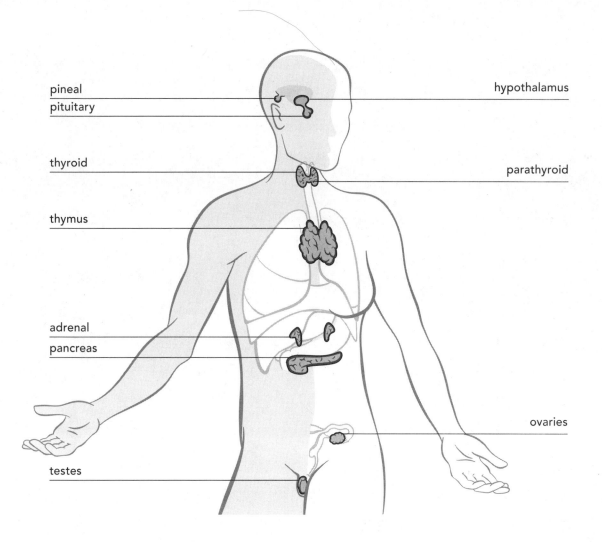

pineal
pituitary
thyroid
thymus
adrenal
pancreas
testes

hypothalamus
parathyroid
ovaries

Key terms

adrenal. A gland above the kidney that produces hormones to regulate heart rate, blood pressure, and other functions.

hormone. A chemical messenger produced by a gland and transported by the bloodstream that regulates specific processes in the body.

parathyroid. An endocrine gland in the neck that produces parathyroid hormone.

pineal gland. A small gland near the center of the brain that secretes melatonin.

pituitary. The endocrine gland at the base of the brain that controls growth and development.

thymus. The lymphoid organ that produces T-cells.

thyroid gland. The gland in the neck that secretes hormones that regulate growth, development, and metabolic rate.

The endocrine system regulates many body functions, including blood production, appetite, reproduction, brain function, sleep cycle, salt-and-water homeostasis, growth, sexual development, and response to stress and injury. Some non-polar, fat-soluble hormones, such as estrogen and progestogen, are released in a pattern set by age and development and their effects are long-lasting. Other polar, water-soluble hormones, such as epinephrine, are released acutely in response to stress, and their actions are short-lived. Hormone imbalance can cause metabolic diseases such as diabetes, hyperthyroidism, and gigantism. Hormone levels are often measured to determine if a disease is present.

The nervous and endocrine systems integrate at the hypothalamus. The nervous system receives signals from the sensory system and uses electrical impulses to send signals to the hypothalamus to activate the pituitary. The pituitary then sends releasing hormones to other glands in the body that controls their hormone production. Hormones are made at the gland and released directly into the circulatory system and are received by the target cell or organ by hormone-specific receptors. Generally, the endocrine system acts more slowly than the nervous system and the effects last longer than nervous system impulses. The TEAS requires knowledge of the relationship between the nervous and endocrine systems.

S.1.8 Practice problems

1. Which of the following describes the signal employed by the endocrine system?

   A. Electrical

   B. Chemical

   C. Physical

   D. Audio-visual

2. Which of the following is not a gland in the endocrine system?

   A. Pineal

   B. Hypothalamus

   C. Lung

   D. Ovary

3. Describe how a gland sends a message.

S.1.9 *Describe the anatomy and physiology of the genitourinary system.*

The organs in the genitourinary, or urogenital, system function in the excretory process. Some structures, such as the urethra and penis in the male, are also used by the reproductive system. This section of the TEAS will focus on the excretion process and its associated structures. Excretion is a necessary function for salt and water homeostasis and getting rid of wastes. It is important to know how the structures function and their contributions to the process of excretion and reproduction.

The genitourinary system is composed of the kidneys, ureters, urinary bladder, and urethra. Kidneys manufacture urine, which travels through the ureters to the urinary bladder where it is stored until excretion through the urethra. In males, the urethra must pass through the penis, and it can also carry sperm. Females have a much shorter urethra.

Kidneys are primarily responsible for filtering blood, creating urine, stabilizing water balance, maintaining blood pressure, and producing the active form of vitamin D. The functional unit of the kidney is the nephron. The kidney is divided into two major regions: the cortex and the medulla. The glomerulus of the nephron located in the renal cortex filters blood to form a dilute plasma-like filtrate, which is concentrated in the proximal and distal convoluted loops of the renal medulla. There, salt and water are resorbed to make urine, which is released into the collecting duct. The collecting ducts drain into the renal pelvis, which opens into the ureter. Urine is a waste product that contains urea, water, salts, and other excess metabolites.

This objective includes, but is not limited to, the following examples of knowledge, skills, and abilities.

- *Identify specific parts of the genitourinary system.*
- *Demonstrate knowledge of the function of the genitourinary system.*
- *Demonstrate knowledge of the relationship between the cardiovascular system and the genitourinary system.*

kidney

cortex

medulla

ureter

urinary bladder

urethra

Kidneys play a vital role in maintaining blood and blood pressure. The cardiovascular system pumps blood into the kidneys through the renal artery. The pressure of the blood helps the glomerulus filter out wastes and return vital nutrients to the blood through the renal vein. The kidneys also produce renin, a hormone that regulates blood pressure by retaining or removing water and salt. The TEAS will ask how the cardiovascular and genitourinary systems are linked.

Nephron

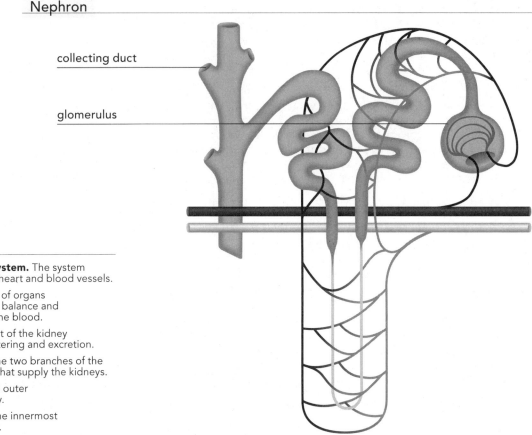

collecting duct

glomerulus

Key terms

cardiovascular system. The system comprised of the heart and blood vessels.

kidneys. The pair of organs that regulate fluid balance and filter waste from the blood.

nephron. The part of the kidney responsible for filtering and excretion.

renal arteries. The two branches of the abdominal aorta that supply the kidneys.

renal cortex. The outer layer of the kidney.

renal medulla. The innermost part of the kidney.

renal pelvis. The center of the kidney where urine collects before moving to the ureter.

renal vein. A vein carrying blood from a kidney to the inferior vena cava.

renin. An enzyme released by the kidney when reduced blood pressure is detected by baroreceptors in aorta and carotid arteries.

urea. The main nitrogenous part of urine.

ureter. The duct that conducts urine from the kidney to the bladder.

urinary bladder. The structure that stores urine in the body until elimination.

urine. Liquid waste matter excreted by the kidneys.

The ureters, urinary bladder, and urethra are parts of the excretory system. The ureters (one for each kidney) are small tubes that carry urine to the urinary bladder, which holds the urine until excretion through the urethra. The urinary bladder is a hollow, muscular organ that holds 400 to 800 mL liquid and has sensors that communicate with the central nervous system. In order for excretion to occur, both the internal and external sphincters of the bladder must relax. The TEAS will ask about the structure and function of the ureters, bladder, and urethra.

s.1.9 Practice problems

1. Which of the following organs functions as part of the genitourinary system to maintain blood pressure?

   A. Heart

   B. Kidney

   C. Urinary bladder

   D. Ureter

2. Which of the following parts of the genitourinary system also transports sperm?

   A. Kidney

   B. Ureter

   C. Urinary bladder

   D. Urethra

3. Which of the following organs filters blood and creates urine?

   A. Heart

   B. Urinary bladder

   C. Lungs

   D. Kidney

S.1.10 *Describe the anatomy and physiology of the immune system.*

The immune system functions like fortifications of a castle to protect the body. For this TEAS task, you'll need to be familiar with the various parts of the immune system and how they contribute to that protection scheme. In particular, you'll need to understand how the immune system relates to the other body systems.

The immune system prevents entry of pathogens through the presence of barriers (much like walls and moats) composed of the skin and secretions such as acid, enzymes, and salt. If the external barriers are breached, there are cells and chemicals that act as soldiers to attack the pathogens. If that barrier fails, then the adaptive immune system specifically identifies, targets, and remembers the pathogen. Visualize the immune system as layers of protection that include barriers to prevent entry, signaling, and targeting. The ultimate function is to protect the body from pathogen attack while allowing harmless molecules to enter the body. The immune system works hand-in-hand with other body systems to transport immune cells, signaling molecules and antibodies throughout the body. Finally, you should be able to recognize diseases caused by failure or overactivity of the immune system.

The immune system protects the body from disease-causing agents. There are two major components of the immune system in vertebrates: **innate** and **adaptive** (or acquired) immune system. Do not confuse the innate immune system with passive immunity. The immune system functions through interactions with several other systems through which pathogens can enter the body via **lymph nodes**. These lymph nodes contain large number of antigen-presenting cells that can trigger the adaptive immune system.

INNATE IMMUNE SYSTEM (nonspecific response)		ADAPTIVE IMMUNE SYSTEM (respond to specific antigens)	
EXTERNAL	INTERNAL	REACTION	PREVENTION
Skin	Antimicrobials	Cytotoxic T-cells kill pathogen	B-cells produce antibodies
Hair	Inflammation		
Mucus	Interferons	Activated by antigen and helper T-cells	
Earwax	Complement		
Secretions (acid, salt, enzymes)	NK lymphocytes	Helper T-cells are activated by APC	
Normal flora	Phagocytes (including APC)		

This objective includes, but is not limited to, the following examples of knowledge, skills, and abilities.

- *Identify specific parts of the immune system.*
- *Demonstrate knowledge of the function of the immune system.*
- *Demonstrate knowledge of the relationship between the immune system and all other systems.*

Key terms

adaptive immune system. A kind of passive or active immunity in which antibodies to a particular antigen are present in the body.

antibody. A blood protein that counteracts a specific antigen.

antigens. Substances on the surfaces of agents that act to identify them, to the body, as being native or foreign.

antigen presenting cell (APC). A cell that displays foreign antigens with major histocompatibility complexes on their surfaces.

antimicrobial. A substance that kills or inhibits growth of micro-organisms with minimal damage to the host.

B-cell. Lymphocytes that mature in bone marrow and make antibodies in response to antigens.

barrier. A divider between parts of the body.

SCIENCE

The innate immune system is a series of nonspecific **barriers**—physical, cellular, and soluble components—that impede pathogens from entering the body or multiplying. External barriers include the physical barrier of the skin and mucus secretions; chemical barriers, such as low pH, salt, enzymes; and cellular barriers of commensal micro-organisms. If the pathogen breaches the barriers and enters the blood or tissues, internal barriers include antimicrobial peptides; interferons that prevent viral replication; complement, which involves the binding of antibodies to the pathogen, inflammation reactions, including fever; "natural killer" (NK) lymphocyte cells that attack host cells that harbor intracellular pathogens; and phagocytic cells that engulf and digest extracellular pathogens. Macrophages and dendritic cells respond to conserved **pathogen-associated molecular patterns** (PAMPs) through **toll-like receptors** and trigger an inflammation or **antigen presentation**.

The adaptive immune system responds by remembering signature molecules, called antigens, from pathogens to which the body has previously been exposed. The adaptive immune system's functional cells are **lymphocytes** called T-cells and B-cells. Antigen-presenting cells (APCs) digest pathogens and present the pathogen's antigen signature to "helper" T-cells. When a **helper T-cell** encounters a cytotoxic T-cell that recognizes the same antigen, it produces **cytokines** that activate the **cytotoxic T-cell**. The cytotoxic T-cell then searches out and destroys any cell that contains the pathogen's antigen signature. The helper T-cell also activates B-cells that recognize the pathogen's signature antigen. This induces the **B-cell** to multiply rapidly into secretory cells called **plasma cells**, which produce large amounts of an **antibody** (Ig, or immunoglobulins) that can bind the antigen. If antigen levels subside, plasma cells stop making antibodies and produce **memory cells** that remember the antigen. Re-encounter with an antigen can trigger rapid activation of plasma cells and cytotoxic T-cells.

Passive and **active** immunity distinguish protection through passive introduction of antibodies as a protective agent or its active production by the body. Rapid treatment for snakebite is an example of passive immunity. Vaccination, in which the body produces antibodies in response to the presence of antigen, is active immunity.

Many diseases are caused by immune system malfunction. Underactivity of the immune system can cause components to be ineffective. AIDS is caused by a virus, HIV, which infects helper T-cells and prevents it from activating cytotoxic T-cells and B-cells, preventing the adaptive immune system from operating. Overactive immune systems can target innocuous foreign particles like pollen, causing the body to go into overdrive by producing huge amounts of IgE that trigger histamine release from mast cells, causing **allergies** with sneezing and mucus secretion. Alternately, the immune system can mistakenly target a host molecule as a foreign antigen, leading to **autoimmune disease**.

Key terms, continued

complement. The group of proteins in blood serum and plasma that works with antibodies to destroy particulate antigens.

dendritic cell. Antigen-presenting cells that process antigen material and present it to T-cells.

immunoglobulin. An antibody.

innate immune system. A collection of nonspecific barriers and cellular responses that serve as an inborn first and second line of defense against pathogens.

macrophage. A large white blood cell that ingests foreign material.

memory cell. A lymphocyte that responds to an antigen upon reintroduction.

phagocytosis. Ingestion of particles by a cell or phagocyte.

plasma cell. A white blood cell that produces a single type of antibody.

T-cell. White blood cells that mature in the thymus and participate in immune response.

S.1.10 Practice problems

1. Which of the following are innate immune system cells that attack host cells harboring an intracellular pathogen?

   A. Natural killer cells

   B. Cytotoxic T-cells

   C. Plasma cells

   D. Dendritic cells

2. Which of the following is a nonspecific immune response?

   A. Antibody secretion by plasma cells

   B. Cytokine secretion by T-cells

   C. Antigen recognition by B-cells

   D. Cytokine-mediated inflammation

3. Sort the following terms as innate or adaptive immune system components: lymphocytes, B-cells, leukocytes, monocytes, dendritic cells, NK cells, complement, inflammation, phagocytosis, cytotoxic T-cells, plasma cells, memory cells, antibodies, Toll-like receptors, interferons, PAMPs, antimicrobial proteins, physical barriers, Helper T-cells, chemical secretions, lysozyme.

S.1.11 *Describe the anatomy and physiology of the skeletal system.*

The skeletal system has three main functions: movement, protection, and metabolism. To be successful at this task, you should know the names of the major bones of the human body, particularly those that help with movement, protection, and synthesis of blood cells. Study the structure of bone, including cells involved in bone synthesis and breakdown. You will also want to be familiar with diseases of the skeletal system, such as osteoporosis and arthritis.

The skeletal system is the scaffold against which muscles pull for movement, and it provides articulation and protection for delicate organs. The system is composed of bone, which is an organ that is constantly being reorganized. Bones synthesize blood and immune cells, as well as store calcium, phosphate, and lipids. Bone is a dynamic **tissue** that is made and broken down according to need. It also functions to provide structural, protective, and metabolic needs. Bones come in four major types: long, short, flat, and irregular.

This objective includes, but is not limited to, the following examples of knowledge, skills, and abilities.

- *Identify specific parts of the skeletal system.*
- *Demonstrate knowledge of the function of the skeletal system.*
- *Demonstrate knowledge of the relationship between the skeletal system and the neuromuscular system.*

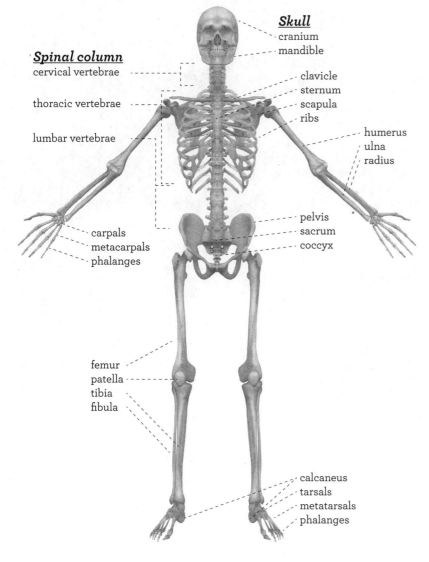

Image credit: beyhes/Getty Images/iStockphoto

Key terms

bone. Hard, calcified material that makes up the skeleton.

brittle bone disease. A group of diseases that affect collagen and result in fragile bones.

canaliculi. Microscoping canals in ossified bone.

cartilage. Tough, elastic connective tissue found in parts of the body such as the ear.

collagen. The primary structural protein of connective tissue.

Haversian canal. Channels in bone that contain blood vessels and nerves.

lamellae. Layers of bone, tissue, or cell walls.

lining cells. Flattened bone cells that come from osteoblasts.

osteoarthritis. Degenerative joint disease.

osteoblasts. Cells that make bone.

osteoclasts. Cells that remove bone.

osteocytes. Bone cells.

SCIENCE

Long bones have long compact hollow shafts containing marrow. The ends are usually made of spongy bone with air pockets. Examples of long bones are humerus, ulna, radius, femur, tibia, and fibula. **Short bones** are wider than they are long. The bones of the toes (metatarsals) and collarbone (clavicle) are short bones. **Flat bones** are not hollow but contain marrow. Examples are the scapula, ribs, and sternum. **Irregular bones** have nonsymmetrical shapes and include the bones of the skull, knee, and elbow. Typically, bones are articulated to other bones through **ligaments** and to muscle through **tendons**. The hyoid bone, which supports the tongue, is the only bone in the body to not connected to other bones, but rather held in place only by muscle. The articulating surfaces of bones are covered in **hyaline cartilage**, which prevents them from grinding against each other. Synovial joints, such as the knee's hinge, also contain lubricating synovial fluid. Synovial joints, such as the pivot, ball-and-socket, and hinge, are usually capable of movement.

There are two main types of bone cells: multinucleate **osteoclasts** and mononucleate **osteoblasts**. Other cells associated with bone originate from osteocytes. Bone is covered by a fibrous sheath called the **periosteum**, which contains nerves and blood vessels. Bone is synthesized in tubular structures called **osteon**, which is composed of calcium and phosphate-rich **hydroxyapatite** embedded in a collagen matrix.

Key terms, continued

osteons. Cylindrical structures that comprise compact bone.

osteoporosis. A disease that causes brittle, fragile bones.

rheumatoid arthritis. A progressive disease that causes joint inflammation and pain.

Volkmann canal. Channels in bone that transmit blood vessels and communicate with Haversian canals.

S.1.11 Practice problems

1. Which of the following cells is involved in mineral resorption from bone?

   A. Osteoclasts

   B. Osteoblasts

   C. Canaliculi

   D. Osteon

2. Which of the following bones articulate at a synovial joint?

   A. Skull bones

   B. Radius and ulna

   C. Bones of the pubis

   D. Humerus and scapula

3. Using the word bank, label the bones of the skeleton.

   calcaneus, carpals, cervical vertebrae, clavicle, coccyx, femur, fibula, humerus, lumbar vertebrae, mandible, metacarpals, metatarsals, patella, pelvis, phalanges (used twice), radius, ribs, sacrum, scapula, skull, sternum, tarsals, thoracic vertebrae, tibia, ulna

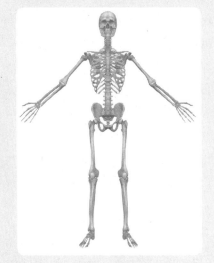

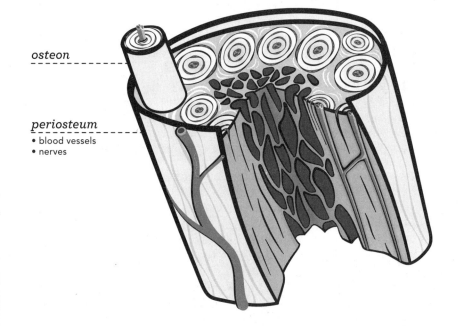

osteon

periosteum
• blood vessels
• nerves

There are several common diseases of bone. Excessive withdrawal of minerals from bone can cause the rigidity of bone to be lost and lead to **osteoporosis**. Cartilage that articulates between joints is damaged in arthritis. **Brittle bone disease** (osteogenesis imperfecta) is due to a genetic defect in the **collagen matrix**, and causes bones to break easily.

Practice problem answers

S.1.1

1. Option C is correct. The cytoskeleton consists of three types of molecules: microtubules, microfilaments, and intermediate filaments. They are involved with cell shape, support, and movement.
   - The Golgi apparatus is responsible for receiving, modifying, and transporting proteins for secretion from the cell.
   - The smooth endoplasmic reticulum lacks ribosomes for protein synthesis. It has three main functions: lipid metabolism, storage of calcium ions, and detoxification of toxins.
   - The cell membrane forms the dynamic outer perimeter of cells, delineating the inside and outside of the cell. It functions in cellular recognition and transport of molecules.

2. Option B is correct. This statement describes the ribs as being further away from the midline of the body.
   - The mouth is below the nose. This would be described as the mouth being inferior to the nose.
   - The patella, or kneecap, is above the shinbone, the tibia. The correct description is that the patella is superior to the tibia.
   - The skin is at the surface of the body and the muscles are away from the surface. The correct description is that the skin is superficial to muscles.

3. Option C is correct. Bone marrow is the site of synthesis of red blood cells in the adult.
   - The liver is involved in the breakdown of red blood cells in the adult.
   - The spleen is involved in the breakdown of red blood cells in the adult.
   - Lymph nodes are filters for the lymphatic system and are not involved in red blood cell production.

S.1.2

1. Option D is correct. Carbon dioxide dissolves in blood to produce H+ and HCO_3^- ions, decreasing pH and increasing acidity. This pH is sensed by the medulla oblongata.
   - Oxygen levels are not sensed by the medulla oblongata.
   - At the end of a sprint, carbon dioxide levels are high, not low.
   - Alkalosis indicates low carbon dioxide levels. This would not occur after a sprint.

2. Option D is correct. Reducing the residual volume of the lung will cause a higher inspiratory volume and an oxygen gradient.
   - Increasing blood flow must be accompanied with increased movement of air to provide optimal gas exchange.
   - Increased oxygen levels will decrease the gradient between the atmosphere and blood, which is less optimal.
   - Reducing alveolar surface area will reduce diffusion and is not efficient.

3. Key:
   - A, 5. Walking pneumonia is caused by mycoplasma infection. Mycoplasma are bacteria lacking cell walls. They infect upper and lower respiratory tract cells and replicate within them. Symptoms are mild, and include headache and cough, but do not require bed rest, hence the name.
   - B, 3. Cystic fibrosis is usually caused by an inherited gene mutation in the chloride transporter in the lung. Due to this disorder, thick mucus accumulates in the lung, causing problems with ventilation and promoting secondary infections.
   - C, 1. Influenza is caused by one of several kinds of RNA-containing viruses in the coronavirus group. This is the only disease caused by a virus in this list.
   - D, 2. Tuberculosis is caused by *Mycobacterium tuberculosis*, which causes lesions in lung tissue. The bacteria wall themselves inside cavities inside the lung to protect from immune attack.
   - E, 4. Mycosis is a fungal disease. The prefix myco- is used in relation to fungus and is applicable to a variety of types of fungi infecting a variety of tissue, including lungs.

S.1.3

1. Option A is correct. Cardiac cells generate electricity in the sinoatrial node and conduct the impulse through the heart to cause muscle contraction.
   - Red blood cells are produced in bone marrow, not in the heart.
   - Cardiac cells do not have immune-protection functions. They contract to pump blood around the body.
   - Cardiac cells do not have excretory functions. Excretory functions are performed by kidney nephrons, skin sweat glands, and lung alveoli.
2. Option B is correct. Vaccines increase the body's recognition of the vaccine antigen, and antibodies should rise following immunization.
   - Red blood cell levels should not increase because vaccines do not contain erythropoietin.
   - Dissolved gas levels should not increase due to immunization.
   - Lymphocytes recognize and respond to antigens. The concentration of leukocytes should remain steady.
3. Option A is correct. The sinoatrial node is the "pacemaker," and it is situated in the top part of the right atrium.
   - The pulmonary vein carries oxygenated blood from the lungs to the heart.
   - The sound is made by the closure of semicircular and atrioventricular valves.
   - The atria are thinner-walled, as they receive blood from veins. Ventricles are thicker-walled, as they pump blood out through the arteries.

S.1.4

1. Option B is correct. Peristalsis is the action that causes food to move in the digestive system, and this increases after food enters the digestive system compared to when there is no food in the digestive system.
   - Pulse rate is usually due to activation of the sympathetic circuit, and the digestive system is controlled by the parasympathetic circuit.
   - Enzymes are required for the digestion of food, thus secretions increase, not decrease.
   - The digestive system is controlled by the parasympathetic nervous system and therefore its activity increases.
2. Option D is correct. In addition to other functions, the liver converts ammonia to urea.
   - The stomach and intestine produce the majority of digestive enzymes.
   - Foods are not filtered through the liver, but the products of digestion are processed in the liver before entering circulation.
   - The liver is not involved in pumping anything around the body.
3. Name:
   - Salivary amylase
   - Pepsinogen
   - Parietal cells
   - Pyloric sphincter
   - Gastrin
   - Cholecystokinin
   - Jejunum
   - Hepatic portal vein
   - Water
   - Rectum

S.1.5

1. Option C is correct.
   - Walking is controlled by voluntary signals.
   - Chewing is controlled by voluntary signals
   - Talking is controlled by voluntary signals
2. Option D is correct.
   - Electrical is how signals move through nerve cells.
   - Kinetic is a type of energy not associated with the synapse.
   - Potential is a type of energy not associated with the synapse.
3. Option B is correct.
   - Fat is responsible for storing energy and protecting nerve cells.
   - Carbohydrates serve as an energy source.
   - Nucleic acids make up DNA.

S.1.6

1. Option B is correct
   - The penis is responsible for delivering sperm.
   - The prostate is responsible for creating fluid to transfer the sperm.
   - The vas deferens are responsible for transferring sperm.
2. Option D is correct
   - The vagina connects the uterus and opening of the body.
   - The cervix is the opening to the uterus from the vagina.
   - The vas deferens are responsible for transferring sperm.
3. Option D is correct
   - Testicles produce sperm.
   - The uterus incubates fetuses.
   - The scrotum holds the testicles.

S.1.7

1. Option D is correct.
   - The dermis is underneath the outer layer.
   - The sudoriferous is a gland in the skin.
   - The sebaceous is a gland in the skin.
2. Option C is correct.
   - Alcohol is excreted through the integumentary system.
   - Minerals are excreted through the integumentary system.
   - Urea is excreted through the integumentary system.
3. Option C is correct.
   - Blood vessel dilation is a cooling process.
   - Sweating is a cooling process.
   - Vitamin D production is neither a cooling or warming process.

S.1.8

1. Option B is correct
   - No electrical impulses are given off by the endocrine system.
   - There are no direct physical connections between an endocrine and its target (except blood, but this is a medium).
   - Hormones do not produce a sound or light show (banter).
2. Option C is correct.
   - The pineal gland produces melatonin.
   - The hypothalamus produces thymosins.
   - The ovary is a gland of the endocrine system
3. Compare your response: The gland synthesizes a hormone, which is released into the blood. The hormone then attaches to a receptor in or on the target gland or tissue to initiate a response

S.1.9

1. Option B is correct.
   - The heart is part of the cardiovascular system.
   - The urinary bladder does not maintain blood pressure.
   - The ureter does not maintain blood pressure.
2. Option D is correct.
   - The kidney filters blood and produces urine.
   - The ureter transports urine from the kidneys to the urinary bladder.
   - The bladder stores urine.
3. Option D is correct.
   - The heart pumps blood.
   - The urinary bladder stores urine.
   - The lungs oxygenate blood.

S.1.10

1. Option A is correct. NK cells sample and attack host cells that harbor intracellular pathogens.
   - Cytotoxic T-cells are a part of the adaptive immune system, not the innate immune system.
   - Plasma cells are antibody-secreting cells and do not attack host cells with intracellular pathogens.
   - Dendritic cells are a type of antigen-presenting cells and do not attack host cells.
2. Option D is correct. Inflammation mediated by cytokines is a nonspecific response to injury or infection.
   - Plasma cells are adaptive immune system B-cells that have been activated to secrete antibodies.
   - T-cells are adaptive immune system cells that are activated by antigen presenting cells.
   - Antigen recognition by the adaptive immune system's B-cells is a specific response to antigen.
3.

Innate Immune System	Adaptive Immune System
Leukocyte	Lymphocytes
Monocytes	B-cells
Dendritic cells	Cytotoxic T-cells
NK cells	Plasma cells
Complement	Memory cells
Inflammation	Antibodies
Phagocytosis	Helper T-cells
Toll-like receptors	
Interferons	
PAMPs	
Antimicrobial proteins	
Physical barriers	
Chemical secretions	
Lysozyme	

S.1.11

1. Option A is correct. Clast means breakdown. Osteoclasts solubilize bone with acid secretions and cause minerals to be resorbed from bone in response to hormonal signals.
   - Osteoblasts make bone by laying down collagen matrix followed by osteon.
   - Canaliculi are small canals in bone through which osteocytes communicate with each other.
   - Osteon is the hydroxyapatite matrix that osteoblasts produce.
2. Option D is correct The ball-and-socket joint of the shoulder is a synovial joint.
   - Skull bones are articulated at sutures and are not movable.
   - The radius and ulna do not move against each other.
   - The pubic bones are fused by cartilage and do not contain synovial joints.

3.

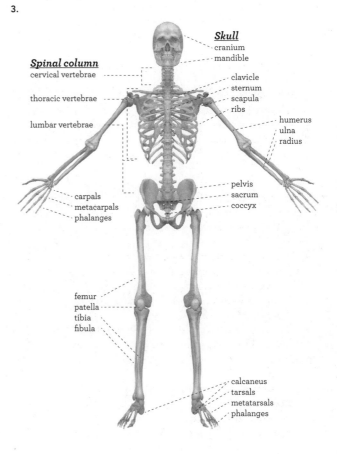

Skull
cranium
mandible

Spinal column
cervical vertebrae
thoracic vertebrae
lumbar vertebrae

clavicle
sternum
scapula
ribs

humerus
ulna
radius

carpals
metacarpals
phalanges

pelvis
sacrum
coccyx

femur
patella
tibia
fibula

calcaneus
tarsals
metatarsals
phalanges

S.2.1 *Describe the basic macromolecules in a biological system.*

Living organisms are composed of a small number of atoms arranged into larger organic molecules. These molecules, called monomers, combine using simple dehydration reactions with other similar molecules to make biological polymers called macromolecules. These macromolecules also function as food groups, and the digestive process breaks down the bonds between monomers by hydrolysis.

You need to understand the basic structure and function of all groups of macromolecules and recognize that their chemical structure makes these possible. Learn to recognize monomer structures, bonds, and polymers, and the reversible reactions that make and break them. Finally, you should be able to recognize the macromolecule category of familiar food items.

Biology and biochemistry textbooks will have a section devoted to macromolecules. You can also look online for overviews and detailed discussions on macromolecules.

Macromolecules are polymers joined together by covalent bonds between the monomeric units. These bonds are made by an endergonic removal of a water molecule (known as dehydration or condensation synthesis). Conversely, these polymers can be broken down by hydrolysis, the addition of water, which breaks the bond and releases monomers and energy. While the process is the same for all macromolecules, the names of the bond between monomers depends on the molecule. There are four types of macromolecules: carbohydrates, lipids, proteins, and nucleic acids.

This objective includes, but is not limited to, the following examples of knowledge, skills, and abilities.

- *Demonstrate knowledge of carbohydrates.*
- *Demonstrate knowledge of lipids.*
- *Demonstrate knowledge of proteins.*
- *Describe how basic macromolecules function in a biological system.*

Formation and breakdown of macromolecule polymers. X represents a monomer and X-X two monomers joined by a covalent bond. OH represents a hydroxyl group.

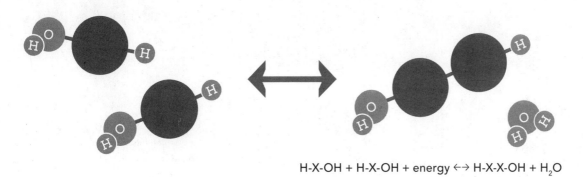

H-X-OH + H-X-OH + energy $\leftrightarrow$ H-X-X-OH + H_2O

Carbohydrate monomers have the general formula $C_nH_{2n}O_n$ where n is typically 3, 4, 5, or 6 carbons long, making triose, tetrose, pentose, or hexose monosaccharides. These monosaccharides are joined together by dehydration synthesis to make disaccharides. Oligosaccharides have longer stretches of linked monosaccharides and polysaccharides, which can be linear or branched, and often have many thousands of monosaccharide units. Carbohydrate functions include structural functions (cellulose, chitin), energy storage (amylose, amylopectin, and glycogen), and recognition molecules (glycoproteins, glycolipids).

Lipids are proteins composed predominantly of hydrogen and carbon, and are often referred to as "fats." Lipids are hydrophobic and therefore help separate aqueous compartments. Lipids such as fats, oils, and adipose store energy efficiently.

SCIENCE

Protein monomers are called amino acids. There are 20 different types of amino acids with different chemical properties based on their side groups, but they all share an amino group and a carboxylic acid group. Amino acids are linked together by peptide bonds and form several types of molecules based on their structure and polarity. Fibrous, hydrophobic molecules like keratin and collagen have hydrophobic amino acids on their surface, are not soluble in water, and are found in structural molecules such as hair and nails. Globular proteins have hydrophilic surface amino acids and are soluble in water (e.g., hemoglobin, antibodies, enzymes). Membrane proteins have a stretch of hydrophobic amino acids sandwiched between layers of hydrophilic amino acids and are found embedded in membranes where they function in transport or signal transfer.

Enzymes are an important class of proteins that catalyze biochemical reactions without being consumed in the reaction. Enzymes speed up reactions by lowering the energy required by the system to initiate the reaction. Reactions can be exergonic (release energy) or endergonic (require energy). Energy in living organisms is typically supplied and released as ATP. Different cell types have a different cocktail of enzymes present based on gene activity, which determines the metabolic function of the cell. Enzyme activity is also regulated by environmental conditions. Enzymes typically have an active site into which the substrate fits and where the catalysis occurs.

The two **nucleic acids** in living systems are deoxyribonucleic acid (DNA) and ribonucleic acid (RNA). DNA is typically a double stranded helix that stores genetic information. It is associated with proteins to form structures called chromosomes located in the nucleus of the cell. DNA contains nucleotides composed of a deoxyribose sugar, one of four nitrogenous bases (adenine, guanine, cytosine, or thymine), and a phosphate molecule. RNA consists of ribonucleotides containing a ribose sugar, a nitrogenous base (adenine, guanine, cytosine, or uracil), and are typically linked in a single-strand molecule. RNA mediates the conversion of the information stored in DNA into the proteins that are encoded by genes. Messenger RNA molecules are copies of the genetic information contained in DNA that is carried to ribosomes where catalytic ribosomal RNA molecules and transfer RNAs work together to make a functional protein. Errors in the precise sequence are referred to as mutations and typically interfere with protein function.

Key terms

carbohydrates. Sugars and starches, which the body breaks down into glucose.

lipids. Fatty acids and their derivatives that are insoluble in water.

macromolecules. A molecule that contains a large number of atoms.

monomers. Molecules that can bond to similar or identical molecules to form a polymer.

nucleic acids. Long molecules made of nucleotides; DNA and RNA.

polymer. A substance composed of similar units bonded together.

proteins. Molecules composed of amino acids joined by peptide bonds.

s.2.1 Practice problems

1. Which of the following is the best description of the characteristics of an enzyme?

    A. Enzymes reduce the initial energy required for a reaction to take place.

    B. The enzyme complement is similar in different cells of the same organism.

    C. An enzyme can operate under a variety of conditions to carry out a reaction.

    D. Enzymes are composed of monomeric units called monosaccharides.

2. Fill in the following table summarizing the properties of macromolecules.

Macromolecule	Monomer	Function(s)	Food example
Proteins		Enzymes Structure Transport Immune	
Carbohydrates		Structure Storage Recognition	
Lipids		Structure Storage	
Nucleic acids		Heredity Regulation	

3. Which of the following is a carbohydrate with structural functions?

    A. Gluten

    B. Lipoprotein

    C. Glycogen

    D. Chitin

4. Define the following terms associated with enzymes.

    A. Catalyst

    B. Activation energy

    C. Specific

    D. Fastidious

    E. Substrate

    F. Exergonic

    G. Endergonic

S.2.2 *Compare and contrast chromosomes, genes, and DNA.*

Hereditary material that passes from one generation to the next is almost always contained in DNA. Genes are DNA-based codes, packaged in units called chromosomes, which guide the production of proteins that directly shape the traits of the actual organism. In this way, offspring inherit traits that allowed their parents to reproduce successfully.

Genes are strung along chromosomes in much the same way that beads are strung on a chain. Genes can be of different lengths and can have structural or regulatory properties. Structural genes are converted into a short-lived RNA message that is decoded by the ribosome and assembled into proteins that go on to build the body. Regulatory genes control the expression of protein-coding genes by turning on or off activity, either directly or through a protein intermediate. In this way, regulatory genes control the expression of different subsets of structural genes in different cell types.

To be successful at this TEAS task, you need to be familiar with terminology. Making flashcards with definitions and sketching figures to represent terms is helpful. There are many resources online that are helpful to visualize these structures.

Deoxyribonucleic acid (DNA) is a macromolecule that contains coded instructions for the body to produce proteins. It is composed of four **nucleotide** letters: A (adenine), T (thymine), G (guanine), and C (cytosine). These letters are arranged in three-letter combinations to make 64 possible "words", called **codons**. A **gene** is a "sentence" made of a specific order of codons that produces a protein. Each codon specifies one amino acid, and these codons instruct ribosomes to assemble the amino acids in a particular order. A **chromosome** is a "chapter" linking sentences with "punctuation marks" that regulate where a gene starts and ends, and which genes are read in which cell.

This objective includes, but is not limited to, the following examples of knowledge, skills, and abilities.

- *Understand the function of chromosomes.*
- *Understand the function of genes.*
- *Understand the function of DNA.*
- *Explain the relationship between chromosomes and genes.*
- *Differentiate among the structures of chromosomes, genes, and DNA.*

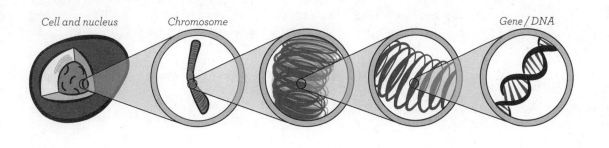

Cell and nucleus   Chromosome   Gene / DNA

DNA is composed of letters paired in a specific order: A always pairs with T on the other strand, and G always pairs with C. Thus **A–T** and **G–C** are referred to as **complementary** bases. The two strands of the DNA **double-helix** "run" in opposite directions. Information is always coded in DNA in the 5' to 3' direction, so this strand is called the "sense" strand. When copying DNA during replication and when transcribing DNA to make messenger RNA, the 3' to 5' "anti-sense" strand is used as template for building a sense strand. In some cases, the two different strands of DNA can actually encode different sentences with different meanings, but only when read in the 5' to 3' direction. The cell can identify the regions that contain embedded information based on punctuation marks embedded in the DNA.

Key terms

chromatid. One of the two duplicates of a chromosome formed during the cell cycle.

chromosome. A structure made of protein and one molecule of DNA.

deoxyribose sugar. The sugar portion of a deoxyribose nucleotide.

deoxyribonucleic acid (DNA). The material that contains genetic information.

gene. A string of DNA that is the basic unit of heredity.

hydrogen bond. A type of non-covalent bond; a weak attraction between a hydrogen atom bound to an electronegative atom and a second highly electronegative atom.

nucleotide. The building block of DNA and RNA.

nucleus. A large organelle within a cell that houses the chromosomes.

phosphate group. A phosphorus atom bound to four oxygen atoms.

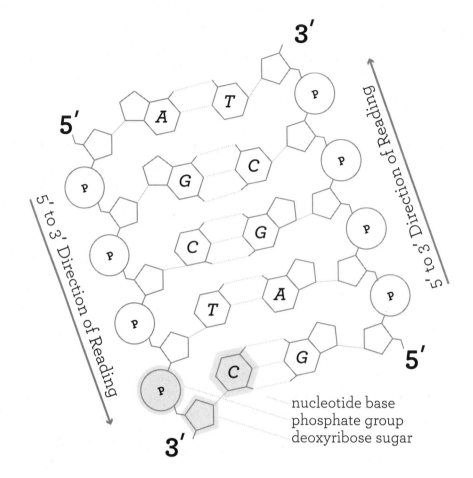

nucleotide base
phosphate group
deoxyribose sugar

Let's look at the detailed structure of a strand of DNA. The nucleotides A, T, G, and C contain the actual information; complementary bases are linked by two **hydrogen bonds** between A and T and three hydrogen bonds between G and C. These weak hydrogen bonds make it possible for the cell to temporarily separate the two strands of the helix in order to read the information. Before a cell divides, chromosomes can be copied to make two identical copies (**chromatids**), which can be separated into two cells or passed on to the next generation.

S.2.2 Practice problems

1. In which of the following directions is DNA read?

   A. Left to right

   B. Top to bottom

   C. 5' to 3'

   D. 3' to 5'

2. A segment of DNA that contains a word made of three nucleotides is referred to as which of the following?

   A. Gene

   B. Codon

   C. Chromosome

   D. Genome

3. Match the letters shown in the figures to their description.

   Nucleotide "letter"

   Codon "word"

   Gene "sentence"

   Chromosome "chapter"

   Genome "book"

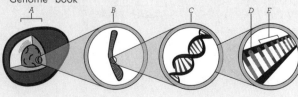

s.2.3 *Explain Mendel's laws of heredity.*

Gregor Mendel was a 19th-century monk who bred peas to study how characteristics are passed from parents to offspring. Through a large number of breeding experiments and statistical analysis of results, Mendel revealed that the patterns underlying inheritance were predictable.

Mendel studied peas, which are diploid, meaning that they contain two copies of each chromosome. Genes for expressed traits (phenotypes) such as plant height are present in two copies, one on each chromosome. The copies of the genes can be identical or different. One variety of gene, called the dominant allele, is expressed in the phenotypic appearance of the plant. The recessive, or nondominant, allele is only expressed if it is present on both the chromosomes. The genotype describes the specific alleles, and the phenotype the plant's external appearance. Mendel's work showed that offspring randomly inherit one chromosome from each parent, male and female. The offspring then express either the dominant or recessive phenotype based on allele composition for the trait. Punnett squares are used to conveniently work out the statistical outcome of these crosses.

For the TEAS, you should understand the difference between inherited and noninherited traits. Inherited traits are passed from parent to offspring through gametes (eggs or sperm). Other traits, such as culturally influenced behavior, are not inherited as part of the genome. Flashcards are useful for memorizing terminology and definitions. Practice drawing Punnett squares to solve simple inheritance problems for both monohybrid and dihybrid ratios. You can find more information on Mendelian inheritance in textbooks and online.

Mendelian inheritance involves studying three generations of pea plants: the **parental** generation (P) which are outcrossed; the first generation of offspring (**filial 1** or F1) which are self-crossed; and the second generation of offspring (**filial 2** or F2), which are subjected to statistical analysis. Parents are chosen to have pure breeding **traits**, one dominant and one recessive. This means that the genome of one parent contains two **alleles** for the **dominant** trait (homozygous dominant genotype) and the other parent has two alleles for the **recessive** trait (homozygous recessive genotype). Dominant alleles are represented by the capital letter for the trait **phenotype** (purple = P), and the recessive allele (white) is represented by the corresponding lowercase letter (p).

Monohybrid inheritance (also known as Mendel's First Law, or the Law of Segregation) refers to the inheritance of a single trait, such as flower color. The parents are **homozygous dominant** (genotype PP; phenotype purple) or homozygous recessive (genotype pp; phenotype white). Because the parents make haploid gametes containing only one chromosome (ovules from the female and pollen from the male), the dominant parent's gametes all have the dominant **P** allele, and the recessive parent's gametes all have the recessive **p** allele. The F1 offspring is produced from a fertilized ovule containing one P and one p allele. This condition of having two different alleles on the two chromosomes is called **heterozygous**, but the phenotype of the F1 offspring is purple. This is because the dominant allele, P, is expressed when it is present. The phenotype of the F2 offspring are analyzed and show a 3:1 monohybrid ratio of purple to white flowers.

This objective includes, but is not limited to, the following examples of knowledge, skills, and abilities.

- *Describe the differences between a dominant and a recessive trait.*
- *Explain how gene pairs are inherited from parents.*
- *Use a Punnett square to predict traits of offspring.*
- *Describe the difference between inheritable and noninheritable traits.*

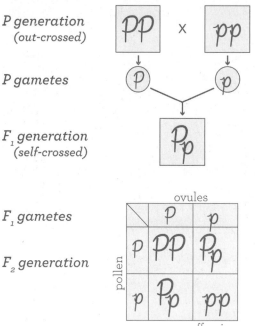

SCIENCE

Key terms

dihybrid cross. A cross between parents heterozygous at two specific genes.

dominant. Refers to the most powerful trait or the allele for that trait.

genotype. The genetic makeup of an individual.

inheritance. Transmission of characteristics to offspring.

Mendelian inheritance. Inheritance of traits that follow Gregor Mendel's two laws and the principle of dominance.

monohybrid cross. A cross between parents heterozygous at one specific gene.

non-Mendelian inheritance. Inheritance of traits that do not follow Mendelian patterns of inheritance.

phenotype. Physical appearance of a trait formed by genetics and environment.

recessive. Refers to traits that are masked if dominant alleles are also present; also refers to the allele for that trait.

Dihybrid inheritance (also known as Mendel's Second Law, or the Law of Independent Assortment) examines the simultaneous inheritance of two separate traits, such as flower color (purple, white) and plant height (tall, dwarf), present on two different sets of chromosomes. Purebred, homozygous parents (phenotypes tall/purple vs. dwarf/white) are out-bred. Gametes produced by the parents have one copy of each gene, and the F1 offspring will be grown from seeds that contain heterozygotes for each gene (TtPp). The phenotype is dominant, and all the plants will be tall with purple flowers. The F1 generation is self-crossed, and pollen is used to fertilize ovules from the same plant. The gametes (pollen or ovule) that are formed must have one allele for each gene. Random combination results in the gametes containing PT, pT, Pt, or pt genotypes. These pollen and ovule gamete genotypes can be used in a Punnett square to study the phenotype outcome for the F2 generation. Examination of the figure to the left gives a pictorial representation of the results: 9 dominant phenotype for both traits; 3 dominant for one trait but recessive for the second; 3 recessive for the first trait but dominant for the second; and 1 recessive for both traits. Thus, **9:3:3:1** is referred to as the **dihybrid ratio**.

Finally, **non-Mendelian** inheritance occurs when there are factors other than dominant/recessive in play. This is not the same as **non-inheritable** traits. Mendelian ratios occur when simple dominance-recessive relationship exists between two alleles; non-Mendelian inheritance is due to factors such as multiple alleles (e.g., blood groups A, B, and O), incomplete dominance-recessive relationships that lead to an intermediate (e.g., pink flowers), co-dominance (AB blood group), and interactions between genes called epistasis. If the 3:1 or 9:3:3:1 relationship is not obtained when the F2 phenotypes are analyzed, it is indicative of non-Mendelian inheritance.

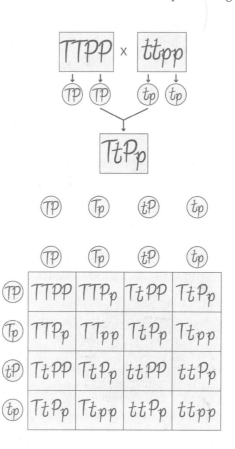

s.2.3 Practice problems

1. The F2 phenotypes of a dihybrid cross show a repeated outcome of 9:3:4 dominant to recessive phenotypes across several experiments. This ratio should be considered which of the following?

   A. Expected monohybrid ratio

   B. Expected dihybrid ratio

   C. Non-inheritable trait being observed

   D. Non-Mendelian ratio being observed

2. A monohybrid cross of a plant with an unknown genotype is carried out with a homozygous recessive plant. The offspring show a 1:1 distribution of dominant:recessive phenotype. The unknown plant was which of the following?

   A. Homozygous recessive

   B. Heterozygous

   C. Homozygous dominant

   D. Showing non-Mendelian inheritance

3. Use the word bank provided to fill in the blanks in the paragraphs below.

   F2, RY, phenotype, ry, monohybrid, F1, homozygous dominant, analyzed, genotype, dominant, parental, two, independent assortment, rY, gene, 3:1, Ry, homozygous recessive, 9:3:3:1, four, dominant-recessive, heterozygous

   __ inheritance depends on the presence of two alleles showing a simple ___ relationship. In the case of this inheritance of one __ with two alleles, the __ generation is analyzed and shows a ratio of __ dominant: recessive phenotypes. F1 plants in this case show dominant __ and heterozygous __.

   Dihybrid ratios relate to the presence of __ genes, and therefore __ alleles. Gametes always contain one allele of each type; thus dihybrid inheritance is governed by the Mendel's Law of __. For example, gametes from a plant with the genotype RrYy will produce the gametes __, __, __, and __. When two heterozygous __ plants are crossed, the F2 offspring are found in the ratio __, also known as the dihybrid ratio.

   In both cases, the __ generation consists of purebred ___ and __ plants; the F1 generations have __ phenotype and __ genotype and the F2 generation's phenotype is __.

S.2.4 *Recognize basic atomic structure.*

The atom is the fundamental constituent of matter that retains the properties of an element. As such, the atom is the smallest unit that has a unique identity. There are 118 elements arranged in the periodic table with increasing proton number, from hydrogen to uranium. While atoms have distinct properties, all are composed of the same three fundamental particles: protons, neutrons, and electrons.

To be successful in this TEAS topic, it is important to understand the structure of an atom and the arrangement of electrons that determine an atom's chemical properties. Atoms undergo chemical reactions by gaining or losing electrons to achieve stability. An atom's properties can be inferred by its position on the periodic table, which relates to the number of valence electrons in its outermost shell. Atoms can lose, gain, or share electrons to make a variety of chemical bonds of varying strengths and properties. Familiarize yourself with the periodic table, get comfortable with identifying the valence of an atom based on its position, and infer the number and type of bonds that an atom would make.

All atoms have a similar structure of a central nucleus containing positively charged **protons** and neutral **neutrons** with negatively charged **electrons** orbiting the nucleus. The negative electrons are held in orbit by their attraction to the positively charged particles in the nucleus and increase in energy with distance from the nucleus. The numbers of neutrons in different atoms of the same element can vary, and these atoms are called **isotopes**.

Subatomic particles have masses and charges related to their identity. The number of protons gives the atomic number of an atom. The number of protons plus neutrons gives the atomic mass of the atom. Atoms are neutral and have equal numbers of protons and electrons.

This objective includes, but is not limited to, the following examples of knowledge, skills, and abilities.

- *Label the parts of the atom.*
- *Know the basic structure of the atom.*
- *Describe an ion.*
- *Using a periodic table, identify the number of electrons and protons.*

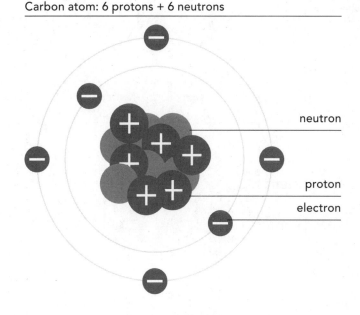

Carbon atom: 6 protons + 6 neutrons

neutron

proton

electron

Subatomic particles	CHARGE	MASS *(atomic mass units)*
Proton	+1	1
Neutron	0	1
Electron	-1	0

The periodic table arranges atoms by increasing **atomic number** (number of protons). Atoms are neutral, so the number of protons equals the number of orbiting electrons. The atomic number is shown as an integer in the periodic table. To identify the number of electrons/protons, look at the integer shown with the element. **Atomic masses** on the periodic table are shown in decimal form to account for the natural abundance of the element's various isotopes.

Because atomic properties are cyclic, the **periodic table** is arranged to highlight these shared properties, grouping similar atoms into vertical columns. Atoms with similar properties have the same number of **valence** (bonding) electrons. Depending on the number of the period, there are different numbers of orbitals that can accommodate different electron numbers. Note that an "s" orbital can accommodate a maximum of two electrons at a time.

Periods represent large electron "highways" with multiple orbital "lanes." For example, the lower energy Period 1 has one "s" orbital with a maximum of 2 electrons allowed. Period 2 has two orbitals: "s" and "p." The "s" orbital can only accommodate 2 electrons, but "p" can accommodate 6 electrons. Therefore, Period 2 can contain a maximum of 8 electrons.

Key terms

anion. A negatively charged ion.

atom. The most basic complete unit of an element.

cation. A positively charged ion.

covalent bond. A chemical bond in which electron pairs are shared between atoms.

electron. A negatively charged atomic particle.

group. A column of elements in the periodic table.

ion. A positively or negatively charged atom or molecule.

ionic bond. The bond between two oppositely charged ions.

Relationship between periods, orbitals, and electrons

PERIOD NUMBER	1	2	3	4
ORBITAL NAMES	s	s	s	s
		p	p	p
			d	d
				f
MAXIMUM NUMBER OF ELECTRONS	s=2	s=2	s=2	s=2
		p=6	p=6	p=6
			d=18	d=18
				f=32

Periodic table of elements

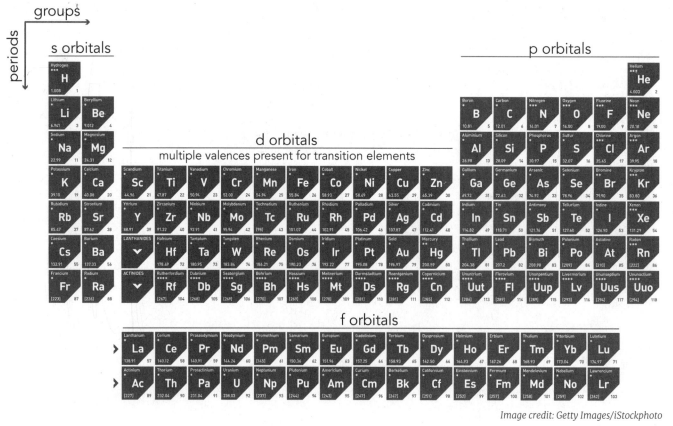

Image credit: Getty Images/iStockphoto

Valence electrons are in the outermost shell of an atom, and participate in chemical reactions (or bonding). Because atoms are most stable when they have a full valence shell like noble gases, all atoms pursue noble gas stability. They gain or lose electrons to do so, forming charged atoms called **ions**. Gaining electrons typically happens in atoms with valences greater than 4, and losing electrons typically happens in atoms with valence less than 4. Observe that all the elements in group 15 will gain 3 electrons and become **negatively charged ions (anions)**. Electrons are donated by atoms that prefer to lose electrons, becoming **positively charged ions (cations)**. Bonds that are formed by transfer of electrons between atoms are called **ionic bonds**, and compounds with **ionic bonds** are soluble in water and conduct electricity.

Atoms can share electrons to achieve stability. For example, two oxygen (O) atoms have 6 valence electrons each. If they each shared 2 electrons, they would both resemble neon in their electron number. This is simpler to understand when visualized. It takes 2 electrons to make one bond, so there are two bonds between the O atoms in O2. These shared bonds are **covalent bonds**. They are typically formed between two p–block elements.

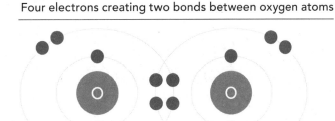

Four electrons creating two bonds between oxygen atoms

Key terms (continued)

neutron. An atomic particle with no electric charge.

orbital. An area around the nucleus where an electron can be found.

period. One of seven horizontal rows in the periodic tables.

periodic table. The table of elements expressed as columns and rows.

proton. A positively charged atomic particle.

valence electron. An electron in an outer orbital that can form bonds with other atoms.

S.2.4 Practice problems

1. Using the information provided in the table, fill in the empty slots.

Element	Proton number	Neutron number	Electron number	Atomic number	Atomic mass (amu)
H	1				1
Mg	12	12			
Mn			25		54
C	6	6			
Ne	10	10			
Pt				78	195
Cl	17	18	17		
Rh		58			103
K			19		59
He	2	2	2		

2. A period in the periodic table represents which of the following?

   A. Shared atomic properties

   B. Increasing energy levels

   C. Decreasing valence electrons

   D. Shared neutron numbers

3. A chemical bond between two atoms contains which of the following?

   A. One electron

   B. Two electrons

   C. Fused atomic nuclei

   D. Electron and proton fusion

4. Match the terms with the definitions.

   _ Cation

   _ Anion

   _ Electron

   _ Neutron

   _ Proton

   A. Negatively charged atom

   B. Positively charged subatomic particle

   C. Neutral subatomic particle

   D. Positively charged atom

   E. Negatively charged subatomic particle

S.2.5 Explain characteristic properties of substances.

This objective includes, but is not limited to, the following examples of knowledge, skills, and abilities.

- *Demonstrate knowledge of density.*
- *Demonstrate knowledge of properties of water (e.g., solubility, cohesion, adhesion).*
- *Identify a substance using characteristics from a chart of given properties.*
- *Compare and contrast osmosis and diffusion.*

Individual substances have unique properties that allow them to be distinguished from other substances. In order to be successful in this TEAS task, recognizing physical characteristics such as density, melting point, boiling point, and polarity are necessary. This task requires a proficient understanding of the characteristics of common substances, particularly those of water. TEAS questions for this task could require you to interpret a data table or distinguish between different properties, so it's important to be well-versed in the most important concepts.

All substances have physical and chemical properties. Physical properties refer to observed properties of the substance and those that can change the state without changing the identity of the substance. An example is boiling liquid water. The steam (vapor) that is produced is a gaseous state of water with the same molecular formula as liquid water. The vapor can be condensed to form liquid water once again. Other physical properties include density, melting point, boiling point, malleability, specific heat capacity, and conductivity. Intensive physical properties (e.g., boiling point, melting point, luster) do not depend on the amount of the substance present. Extensive physical properties (e.g., mass and volume) can change depending on the amount of matter present.

Chemical properties depend on the chemical reactivity of the substance. When a substance chemically reacts with another substance, it results in formation of a new substance with a different composition and identity. A sugar cube can be cut in half, changing the volume of each half (an extensive physical property). But if the sugar cube is burned, the sugar combines with oxygen, converting sugar to the new substances carbon dioxide and water.

Atomic Number	Symbol	Name	First ionization energy (kJ/mol)	Electro-negativity	Melting point (K)	Boiling point (K)	Density (g/cm³)	Atomic radius (pm)
1	H	hydrogen	1312	2.2	14	20	0.000082	32
2	He	helium	2372			4	0.000164	37
3	Li	lithium	520	1.0	454	1615	0.534	130
4	Be	beryllium	900	1.6	1560	2744	1.85	99
5	B	boron	801	2.0	2348	4273	2.34	84
6	C	carbon	1086	2.6				75
7	N	nitrogen	1402	3.0	63	77	0.001145	71
8	O	oxygen	1314	3.4	54	90	0.001308	64
9	F	fluorine	1681	4.0	53	85	0.001553	60
10	Ne	neon	2081			24	27	0.000825	62

Physical properties can be used to identify substances. For example, density is the ratio of mass to volume. This ratio is not dependent on the size of the sample, but rather the unique structure of the substance. This means that a sample of water has a density of 1 gram per cubic centimeter ($1 g/cm^3$) independent of the sample size. TEAS tasks might ask test takers to identify substances using a chart of physical properties. For example, using the data table provided, it can be determined that an element with a melting point of 63 K and a boiling point of 77 K is nitrogen.

Water has several unique properties. It is a polar molecule, which means it has negatively charged (oxygen end) and positively charged (hydrogen end) sides. The polarity of water allows it to form hydrogen bonds and demonstrate both cohesive and adhesive properties. The cohesiveness of water allows it to travel through small capillaries without using energy. Cohesiveness also creates surface tension by creating a tight-knit layer of water molecules on the surface of any body of water. Breaking up the multitude of hydrogen bonds between water requires a lot of energy, so water is said to have high specific heat and high heat of vaporization. Ice floats on water because it has lower density than water. The adhesiveness of water allows it to stick to other molecules. Water is also considered the universal solvent, meaning many substances dissolve in water.

Diffusion and osmosis are key processes for the transport of molecules through substrates and across membranes. Diffusion is a generic term for any substance moving from areas of high concentration to areas of low concentration. This is best exemplified by spraying perfume in a room: The perfume will at first be very concentrated where it was sprayed but over time, the perfume diffuses through the air until the concentration is the same in all areas of the room. Osmosis is a specific type of diffusion pertaining to water moving passively across a membrane through pores made of aquaporin proteins. Water moves from regions of high to regions of low water concentration without the use of energy. To move from regions of low to high concentrations, energy must be used.

Key terms

boiling point. The temperature at which a liquid boils and turns into vapor.

chemical properties. Characteristics of a material that present during a chemical reaction or chemical change.

density. The amount of mass per volume.

diffusion. The passive movement of substances from areas of high concentration to areas of low concentration.

extensive properties. Properties that depend on the size of the sample of a substance.

intensive properties. Properties that do not depend on the size of the sample of a substance.

malleability. The ability of a metal to be shaped.

melting point. The temperature at which a solid changes to a liquid.

nonpolar. A type of covalent bond in which two atoms share electrons at equal distances from their atomic nuclei.

osmosis. Passage of fluid through a membrane.

physical properties. Observable properties of matter.

polar. A type of covalent bond in which two atoms share electrons that are not at equal distances from their atomic nuclei. If the geometry of the molecule does not equalize the partial charges created by the polar covalent bond, the region of partial charge remains unbalanced, and the molecule is considered polar.

specific heat capacity. The amount of energy needed to change the temperature of 1 gram of a substance by 1° Celsius.

SCIENCE

S.2.5 Practice problems

1. Which of the following is the density of a substance that has a mass of 26.5 g and a volume of 3.4 cm³?

   A. 0.13 g/cm³

   B. 0.68 g/cm³

   C. 7.8 g/cm³

   D. 90 g/cm³

2. Which of the following is true about osmosis?

   A. Osmosis is the movement of water across a membrane.

   B. Osmosis is movement from a low concentration to a high concentration.

   C. Osmosis requires a large amount of energy to move water.

   D. Osmosis pertains to all molecules moving across a membrane.

3. Use the table on the previous page to determine the boiling point, melting point, and density of oxygen.

S.2.6 *Compare and contrast changes in states of matter.*

This objective includes, but is not limited to, the following examples of knowledge, skills, and abilities.

- *Describe the states of matter.*
- *Demonstrate knowledge of the movement of molecules in the states of matter.*
- *Discriminate among the different phases of matter.*
- *Explain changes between states of matter (e.g., melting, freezing, evaporation, condensation).*

Key terms

boiling. The transition of liquid to gas when a substance has acquired enough thermal energy.

condensation. The transition of a gas to a liquid.

critical point. The temperature at which the liquid and gas phases of a substance have the same density.

deposition. The transition of a substance from gas to solid without passing through the liquid state.

evaporation. The transition of liquid to gas that happens with or without the substance acquiring enough thermal energy to reach its boiling point.

freezing. The transition of a liquid to a solid.

gas. A state of matter that does not have a definite volume or shape and is highly compressible.

liquid. A state of matter that has definite volume but not definite shape.

melting. The transition of a solid to a liquid.

phase diagram. A graph of physical states of a substance under varying temperature and pressure.

solid. A state of matter that retains its shape and density when not contained.

sublimation. The transition of a substance from solid to gas without passing through the liquid state.

triple point. The temperature and pressure at which solid, liquid, and vapor phases of a pure substance coexist.

Matter can exist in different states determined by environmental conditions. In this TEAS task, it is important to distinguish among states of matter and explain how the movement of the molecules is related to the state of matter. In order to be successful, it will be necessary to explain the transition of matter between phases. The TEAS uses examples from different substances, so knowing how the processes work is important.

Molecules make up all matter. Matter exists in four phases: solid, liquid, gas, and plasma. TEAS focuses on questions about solids, liquids, and gases. Above absolute zero (0 K or –273 °C), molecules are in constant motion. According to the Kinetic Molecular Theory, molecular motion changes as heat is added or removed. Heat overcomes the forces that hold matter together. As the temperature of a substance increases, the intermolecular forces that hold the molecules together are broken, causing the molecules to move away from each other. The amount of heat required for a phase change will not break the bonds within a molecule. In solids, the molecules are packed together in a tight, orderly pattern; there is vibrational motion but no translational motion experienced by the molecules. The molecules in liquids are less ordered, and exhibit both translational and vibrational motion. Gas molecules are rapidly moving and spread far apart.

The phase of a substance depends on two conditions: temperature and pressure. Increasing temperature has a tendency to move the particles of matter apart, and increasing pressure has a tendency to pack them closer together. In the phase diagram for carbon dioxide, the temperature and pressures for solid, liquid, and gaseous carbon dioxide are shown. At the triple point, solid, liquid, and gas coexist; above the critical point, liquid, and gas coexist.

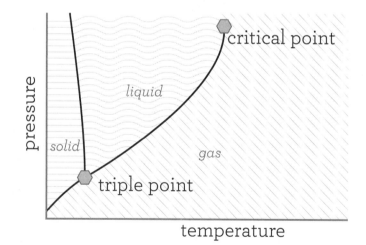

Solid matter has definite volume and shape. Liquid matter has definite volume but no definite shape, meaning that it will conform to the shape of the container. Gas has no definite volume or shape. Gases are highly compressible and subject to changes in volume, but liquids and solids are generally non-compressible.

A change from solid to liquid (melting) requires an addition of heat, which causes the molecules to become more energized and increases their vibrational and translational motion. Adding heat is also required to change matter from liquid to gas (boiling). Removing heat from matter is required to change gas to liquid (condensation) or liquid to solid (freezing). An unusual phase change is the direct conversion of solids to gas called sublimation. In deposition, the reverse phase change from gas directly to solid occurs. These occur at room temperature with the element iodine and the molecule carbon dioxide. TEAS tasks might ask how heat is related to phase changes.

s.2.6 Practice problems

1. Which of the following phase changes requires the addition of heat?

   A. Freezing

   B. Condensation

   C. Melting

   D. Deposition

2. Which of the following is true of gases?

   A. Gases have definite shape and volume.

   B. Gases have no definite shape, but they have definite volume.

   C. Gases have a definite shape, but no definite volume

   D. Gases have no definite shape and no definite volume

3. Place the states of matter in order from least molecular motion to greatest molecular motion.

S.2.7 *Describe chemical reactions.*

This objective includes, but is not limited to, the following examples of knowledge, skills, and abilities.

- *Identify covalent and ionic bonds.*
- *Identify simple chemical reactions.*
- *Describe how conditions affect chemical reactions (e.g., pressure, concentration, temperature).*
- *Describe how catalysts (enzymes) affect chemical reactions.*
- *Knowledge of basic molecules (e.g., H_2O, NaCl, CO_2, O_2, $C_6H_{12}O_6$, KCl).*
- *Describe acids and bases in terms of pH balance.*

This TEAS task will focus on aspects of chemistry. Chemical reactions are occurring constantly in nature by creating and breaking bonds between elements and compounds. These reactions occur at varying rates with changing conditions.

Chemical bonds occur when two or more atoms have interactions between electrons. Ionic bonds can only form when the elements involved have a large difference in electronegativity, such as exists between metals and nonmetals. This difference allows for the donation of electrons from one element to the other. These elements then become ions or charged atoms. Metals tend to become positively charged cations, and nonmetals become negatively charged anions. Covalent bonds require the sharing of electrons and occur between two nonmetals. In covalent bonds, there is not a sufficient difference in electronegativity to gain or lose electrons. However, differences in electronegativity within a covalently bonded molecule cause them to be polar or nonpolar. You should be able to recognize metals and nonmetals using a periodic table.

Chemical reactions are represented by chemical equations. Chemical equations have a basic pattern: reactants, reaction sign showing the direction of the reaction ($\rightarrow$), and products. The formation of salt is an example of a chemical equation: $2Na + Cl_2 \rightarrow 2NaCl$. Chemical equations must be shown as balanced equations, meaning there must be the same number of each element on both sides. There are five basic chemical reactions: synthesis, decomposition, single replacement, double replacement, and combustion. TEAS tasks will ask about bonds and chemical reactions.

Reaction rates can be altered by changing certain conditions: pressure, concentrations of reactants and substrates, temperature, and the presence of catalysts can be altered to slow down or speed up reactions. All of these conditions can be applied to the equation to assess the rate of reaction. If temperature rises, then the rate of an endothermic reaction (where heat is a reactant) will increase, but that of an exothermic reaction (where heat is a product) will slow down. Increasing the concentration of reactants increases the probability that reactants will come in contact with each other, therefore increasing the likelihood of breaking or creating a bond; if product concentration is increased, the reaction will slow down. Catalysts act by lowering the activation energy required for a chemical reaction to occur, and so they can speed up reactions that would otherwise be extremely slow to occur in nature. The catalyst does not change during the reaction and is regenerated. In biological systems, catalysts are called enzymes. TEAS tasks require knowledge of reaction rates and conditions that can change those rates.

Acids and bases have distinct chemical interactions. Acids either donate H+ ions or accept OH- ions, and they have pH less than 7 on the pH scale. Bases either donate OH- ions or accept H+ ions, and they have a pH greater than 7 on the pH scale. Acids and bases react with each other to produce water and salt. When the proper amount of acid and base is used, then the system becomes neutral with a pH of 7. TEAS tasks require knowledge of acids, bases, and the pH scale.

A general knowledge of compounds is necessary to complete TEAS tasks. Salts including $NaCl$ (sodium chloride), KCl (potassium chloride), and $NaBr$ (sodium bromide) could be included on the test. In order to be successful on the TEAS, it will be important to know the formulas and names of covalent compounds such as H_2O (water), CO_2 (carbon dioxide), and O_2 (oxygen in its natural state). The last compounds to study are organic molecules $C_6H_{12}O_6$ (glucose) and C_2H_6O (ethanol).

Key terms

acid. A substance with a pH less than 7.

base. A substance with a pH greater than 7.

catalyst. A substance that increases the rate of a chemical reaction without undergoing permanent chemical change.

chemical equation. Mathematic representation of a chemical reaction.

compound. A substance made of two or more elements.

element. Pure substances that cannot be broken into simpler substances.

enzyme. A substance produced by a living thing that acts as a catalyst.

metal. A substance that is a good conductor of electricity and heat, forms cations by loss of electrons, and yields basic oxides and hydroxides.

nonmetal. Any element or substance that is not a metal.

organic molecule. A molecule found in a living thing that contains carbon.

pH. The measure of acidity or alkalinity.

salt. A chemical compound formed from the reaction of an acid with a base, with at least part of the hydrogen of the acid replaced by a cation.

s.2.7 Practice problems

1. Which of the following substances contains an ionic bond?

   A. CO

   B. NO_2

   C. SO_4

   D. CaO

2. In the following equation, what are the reactants?

   $AgNO_3 + NaCl \rightarrow AgCl + NaNO_3$

   A. $AgNO_3$, NaCl, AgCl, $NaNO_3$

   B. $AgNO_3$, NaCl

   C. NaCl, AgCl

   D. AgCl, $NaNO_3$

3. True or False: A substance with a pH of 3.7 is considered a base.

Practice problem answers

S.2.1

1. Option A is correct. Enzymes reduce activation energy, which is the energy required to initiate a reaction.
   - Enzymes are transcribed and translated from genes, but the complement of enzymes in different cells is different and based on the cell's function.
   - Enzymes are highly reactant and product-specific. They work under a very narrow set of conditions, depending on the enzyme.
   - Enzymes are proteins and are composed of monomers called amino acids. Some RNA molecules have catalytic activity, but they are referred to as ribozymes and have ribonucleotide monomers.

2. Table summarizing the properties of macromolecules.

Monomer	Function(s)	Food example
MACROMOLECULE: PROTEINS		
Amino acids	Enzymes: catalysis Structure: muscle, keratin Transport: hemoglobin Immune: antibodies	Meat Egg white
MACROMOLECULE: CARBOHYDRATES		
Monosaccharides	Structure: cellulose, chitin Storage: glycogen, amylose Recognition: glycoproteins, glycolipids	Bread Potatoes
MACROMOLECULE: LIPIDS		
Fatty acids	Structure: phospholipids Storage: adipose	Oils Butters
MACROMOLECULE: NUCLEIC ACIDS		
Nucleotides	Heredity: DNA, RNA Regulation: RNA	No specific food example; found in small amounts in all foods

3. Option D is correct. Chitin is a nitrogen-containing carbohydrate that is an important constituent of cells walls of fungi and animal exoskeletons.
   - Gluten is a protein.
   - Lipoprotein is made of lipids and proteins.
   - Glycogen is the storage form of carbohydrates in animals.

4. Correct definitions
   - Catalyst: Something that speeds up a chemical reaction but is not changed in the process.
   - Activation energy: The energy needed to initiate a chemical reaction.
   - Specific: The observation that an enzyme catalyzes a limited chemical reaction with a specific substrate and product.
   - Fastidious: Requiring narrow environmental conditions.
   - Substrate: The reactant in a chemical reaction.
   - Exergonic: A chemical reaction that releases energy as a product.
   - Endergonic: A chemical reaction that requires energy to occur.

S.2.2

1. Option C is correct. DNA is read from 5′ to 3′
   - There is no left and right in chromosomes.
   - There is no top and bottom in chromosomes.

2. Option B is correct. A codon is a three-nucleotide "word" that codes for an amino acid.
   - A gene is an instructional "sentence" made of codon "words."
   - A chromosome is composed of a length of DNA incorporating a linear arrangement of genes on each strand. A gene is made of codon "words" that link to form a gene "sentence."
   - A genome represents the sum total of all the chromosomal information in the cell.

3. Correct pairs
   - A. Genome "book"
   - B. Chromosome "chapter"
   - C. Gene "sentence"
   - D. Nucleotide "letter"
   - E. Codon "word"

S.2.3

1. Option D is correct. The distorted 9:3:3:1 ratio with the last two numbers being combined to one is a non-Mendelian ratio due to interaction or other interference between genes.
   - An expected monohybrid ratio would be 3:1.
   - A dihybrid ratio is 9:3:3:1.
   - A non-inheritable trait would not necessarily have a ratio that was repeated.

2. Option B is correct. A heterozygous plant with one dominant and one recessive allele would produce gametes with either one dominant or one recessive allele. Crossed to a homozygous recessive plant whose gametes are all recessive, this would yield 50% dominant phenotype and 50% recessive phenotype.
   - A homozygous recessive plant crossed to a homozygous recessive plant would yield 100% recessive phenotypes.
   - A homozygous dominant plant will have two dominant alleles and produce all dominant allele-containing gametes. When crossed with a homozygous recessive plant producing all-recessive gametes, they will produce heterozygous offspring with dominant phenotype.
   - The monohybrid 3:1 ratio is only applicable to the F2 offspring of a heterozygote self-cross.

3. **Monohybrid** inheritance depends on the presence of two alleles showing a simple **dominant-recessive** relationship. In the case of this inheritance of one **gene** with two alleles, the **F2** generation is analyzed and shows a ratio of **3:1** dominant: recessive phenotypes. F1 plants in this case show dominant **phenotype** and heterozygous **genotype**.
   Dihybrid ratios relate to the presence of **two** genes, and therefore **four** alleles. Gametes always contain one allele of each type; thus dihybrid inheritance is governed by the Mendel's Law of **independent assortment**. For example, gametes from a plant with the genotype RrYy will produce the gametes **RY**, **rY**, **Ry**, and **ry**. When two heterozygous **F1** plants are crossed, the F2 offspring are found in the ratio **9:3:3:1**, also known as the dihybrid ratio.
   In both cases, the **parental** generation consists of purebred **homozygous dominant** and **homozygous recessive** plants; the F1 generations have **dominant** phenotype and **heterozygous** genotype and the F2 generation's phenotype is **analyzed**.

S.2.4

1. Correct data

Element	Proton number	Neutron number	Electron number	Atomic number	Atomic mass (amu)
H	1	0	1	1	1
Mg	12	12	12	12	24
Mn	25	30	25	25	55
C	6	6	6	6	12
Ne	10	10	10	10	20
Pt	78	117	78	78	195
Cl	17	18	17	17	35
Rh	45	58	45	45	103
K	19	20	19	19	59
He	2	2	2	2	4

2. Option B is correct. Periods show increasing energy levels. The farther an electron is from the nucleus, the higher its energy.
   - Shared atomic properties are a function of groups, not periods.
   - Valences are shared in atoms lined up in vertical columns. Periods represent increasing energy levels of atomic shells.
   - The periods represent increasing electron numbers, not shared neutron numbers.
3. Option B is correct. A bond is made of two electrons.
   - The atom nuclei stay distinct.
   - Electrons do not fuse with protons in chemical bonds.
4. Matched terms.
   - Cation. Positively charged atom
   - Anion. Negatively charged atom
   - Electron. Negatively charged subatomic particle
   - Neutron. Neutral subatomic particle
   - Proton. Positively charged subatomic particle

S.2.5

1. Option C is correct. This is the correct ratio of mass to volume: 26.5 divided by 3.4.
   - Option A is the inverse of density: 3.4 divided by 26.5.
   - Option B is 26.5 divided by 3.43. This is a common error in which the unit is cubed, but the number is not.
   - Option D is 26.5 multiplied—not divided—by 3.4.
2. Option A is correct.
   - Like diffusion, osmosis is movement from a high concentration to low concentration.
   - Osmosis does not use energy.
   - Osmosis is specific to water.
3. Boiling point: 90 K
   Melting point: 54 K
   Density: 0.001308 g/cm_3

S.2.6

1. Option C is correct. Melting is a phase change from solid to liquid that requires the addition of heat.
   - Freezing is a phase change from liquid to solid that requires a subtraction of heat.
   - Condensation is a phase change from gas to liquid that requires the subtraction of heat.
   - Deposition is a phase change from gas to solid that requires the subtraction of heat.
2. Option D is correct.
   - Solids have a definite shape and volume.
   - Liquids have no definite shape but definite volume.
   - No state of matter has a definite shape and no definite volume.
3. Solid, liquid, gas. Solids are tightly packed and orderly, liquids have less order, and gases have even less order, allowing for more motion.

S.2.7

1. Option D is correct. There is a metal and a nonmetal.
   - In the other options, both elements are nonmetals, making them covalent bonds.
2. Option B is correct.
   - Option A includes all the elements in the equation.
   - Option C has one reactant and one product.
   - Option D includes two products.
3. False. Acids have a pH less than 7, and bases have a pH greater than 7. A substance with a pH of 3.7 is an acid.

S.3.1 *Identify basic scientific measurements using laboratory tools.*

This TEAS section focuses on scientific measurements, scale, and tools. Accuracy in measuring, recording, and diagramming data are important skills. The TEAS will ask questions that include tools and measurements of volume, mass, and length. It will be necessary to understand the numbers and units involved in measuring large and small quantities of objects and substances.

Scientists use the metric system, or SI system, to measure and record data. This system uses base units and prefixes to increase or decrease size. The SI base units for mass, length, and time are kilogram, meter, and second, respectively. The volume of a three-dimensional object has length, width, and height, all of which are measured in length units. Thus, the volume of a container 10 cm × 10 cm × 10 cm is 1,000 cm^3. This volume is more familiarly called a liter.

Prefixes represent sizes of units. For instance 1 kilometer is 1,000 meters, and 1 centimeter is 0.01 meters. The prefixes can be used with any base. So 1 kilometer is 1,000 meters, and 1 centigram is 0.01 grams. The TEAS will cover prefixes including kilo, hecta, deca, deci, centi, and milli.

Measurements

centi. One hundredth

deca. Ten

hecta. One hundred

kilo. One thousand

milli. One thousandth

It is important to determine the most appropriately scaled unit to use when measuring items. Large items with a lot of mass likely would be measured using kilograms. It is more efficient to say a person has a mass of 75 kg than to say a person has a mass of 75,000 grams. To measure the diameter of a dime, it is easier to use millimeters instead of meters. TEAS tasks will ask which scale is most appropriate for measuring familiar objects.

Tool selection will also be part of this section of the TEAS. There are two types of balances used to measure mass: the triple beam balance and electronic balance. The electronic balance is more common due to its ease of use. Several types of glassware can be used to measure the volume of liquids. The most accurate tool in measuring large volumes is a volumetric flask, and small volumes are best measured using a volumetric pipette. Graduated cylinders are familiar, though less accurate, tools for measuring a range of volumes in the laboratory. The volume of solids can be calculated by multiplying the measurements of length, width, and height; these are measured using rulers, meter sticks, or measuring wheels.

The TEAS will ask about the measurement of a diagram or to determine the scale of the diagram. It will be necessary to determine the appropriate tool, read the tool correctly, and determine the scale. TEAS tasks will focus on volume, mass, and length.

This objective includes, but is not limited to, the following examples of knowledge, skills, and abilities.

- *Identify the unit of measurement in a model (e.g., diagram, illustration, photograph).*
- *Identify the numerical value of a measurement of an object.*
- *Select the tool necessary to measure volume, mass, or length of an object.*
- *Choose a scale unit appropriate for the object being measured.*

Key terms

graduated cylinder. A narrow cylinder used to measure liquid volume.

gram. Metric unit of mass.

length. Measurement of distance from end to end.

liter. Measurement of liquid volume.

mass. A measurement of inertia, commonly considered the amount of material contained by an object and causing it to have weight in a gravitational field.

meter. Basic unit of length in the metric system.

SI units. International System of Units based on meters, kilograms, seconds, amperes, Kelvin, candela, and mole. Commonly known as the metric system.

volume. The amount of space something takes up.

volumetric pipette. A device used for precise measurement of small amounts of liquid.

SCIENCE

S.3.1 Practice problems

1. Which of the following is the most appropriate unit to measure the length (distance) between Los Angeles and San Francisco?

   A. Liter

   B. Meter

   C. Kilometer

   D. Centimeter

2. What does the prefix milli mean?

   A. 1,000

   B. 100

   C. 0.01

   D. 0.001

3. Which of the following tools could be used to measure the mass of a sample?

   A. Triple beam balance

   B. Volumetric pipette

   C. Graduated cylinder

   D. Ruler

S.3.2 *Critique a scientific explanation using logic and evidence.*

This objective includes, but is not limited to, the following examples of knowledge, skills, and abilities.

- *Identify a logical conclusion based on evidence provided.*
- *Identify the stated cause in a scientific explanation.*
- *Identify the stated effect in a scientific explanation.*
- *Evaluate evidence that supports a scientific explanation.*

Key terms

bias. Prejudice in favor of an idea.

empirical. Based on observation.

data. A collection of information.

conclusion. An end judgment based on data.

experiment. A scientific procedure to test a hypothesis.

Constructing meaningful conclusions from data is a central idea in practicing scientific thinking. It is vital in understanding the scientific process to analyze evidence and draw logical explanations. It is also an important skill to analyze scientific arguments for evidence. In this TEAS section, it will be necessary to read scientific information, analyze the content, and construct meaning.

Empirical evidence, or evidence generated through experimentation, is a primary feature of science. Scientists collect data, analyze it, and then draw logical conclusions supported by the data. In this process of sense-making, it is important to understand the data and only look for logical explanations stemming from experimentally reproducible data. TEAS tasks might ask that a conclusion be drawn from pieces of evidence.

Conclusions are often presented as cause-and-effect relationships as understood by the scientist. Although these relationships can be difficult to establish conclusively, scientists use this simplified relationship to explain phenomena. Identifying cause and effect in a situation is necessary for completing TEAS tasks.

Conclusions rely on the evidence that supports them. Analyzing the strength of evidence used to support an argument is imperative to understanding the tentativeness of the conclusion. Strong conclusions and theories are produced by reproducible and convincing data. The process of analyzing data can be tedious, but the following points should usually be observed: presence of bias (either intentional or unintentional), controlled setting (changing only one variable at a time), accurate data collection, and replicable results. TEAS tasks might ask that evidence for a conclusion be analyzed.

S.3.2 Practice problems

A researcher collects data on subjects in an experiment over the course of 1 month. Every day at 11 a.m., every subject takes three pills (A, B, C) to control blood pressure. The following data are collected.

Client number	Initial blood pressure (mm Hg)	Final blood pressure (mm Hg)
1	135/95	130/90
2	130/80	115/70
3	140/90	120/80
4	145/95	120/75

1. Which of the following conclusions can be drawn from the data?
   A. Pill A is effective in treating blood pressure.
   B. Blood pressure went down for all subjects.
   C. The pill regimen is effective for the subjects.
   D. 11 a.m. is the correct time to take pills to decrease blood pressure

2. What type of bias is present if clients 1 and 2 were given instructions to not exercise and clients 3 and 4 were given instructions to exercise?

3. Which of the following is the term used to describe a specific experimental condition that is changed to measure its effect?
   A. Data
   B. Variable
   C. Control
   D. Bias

S.3.3 *Explain relationships among events, objects, and processes.*

The natural world—including the human body—is constantly changing. Events such as earthquakes and epidemics affect many people, while specific ailments affect individuals. It is important to distinguish between the magnitude of large- and small-scale events, objects, and processes. This portion of the TEAS focuses on magnitude, causal relationships, and sequences.

The human body has many cells, tissues, and organs. Each unique component comes in different sizes and often is reported with different scales. For example, the diameter of human hair can be measured in micrometers (millionths of a meter), and the height of a human would more commonly be measured in meters. Every measurement will be given with a unit, and it is the unit that identifies the scale (e.g., kilograms, grams, milligrams). It is important to understand the concept of scale for the TEAS.

Causal relationships are difficult to make definite. However, it will be necessary to define the cause and effect from given information in an example. Studies have linked certain causal relationships, such as smoking and emphysema, high blood pressure and vascular disease, and alcohol consumption during pregnancy and fetal alcohol syndrome.

Determining a causal relationship can also mean determining the sequence of events that leads to a consequence. For instance, going to a bar might lead to drinking alcohol, which might lead to driving while intoxicated, which might lead to an accident. In this scenario, the order of events is important. The accident is caused by driving under the influence of alcohol. Another example is overeating leading to obesity, which can lead to health problems such as high blood pressure. The TEAS will ask questions about causal relationships and sequencing.

This objective includes, but is not limited to, the following examples of knowledge, skills, and abilities.

- *Compare the magnitude (e.g., size) of events, objects, and processes.*
- *Determine the causal relationship between events (e.g., smoking and high blood pressure).*
- *Sequence an event or process.*

Key terms

cause. The element that makes something happen.

effect. The result of a cause.

sequencing. Organization of cause and effect relationships.

SCIENCE

S.3.3 Practice problems

1. Which of the following units is most appropriate for measuring the weight of an adult?

   A. Grams

   B. Kilograms

   C. Milligrams

   D. Micrograms

2. Which of the following units is appropriate for measuring the circumference of the Earth?

   A. Kilometers

   B. Meters

   C. Centimeters

   D. Micrometers

3. Which of the following can lead to emphysema, which is a severe respiratory problem?

   A. High-salt diet

   B. Alcohol consumption

   C. Smoking cigarettes

   D. Sleep deprivation

S.3.4 *Analyze the design of a scientific investigation.*

This objective includes, but is not limited to, the following examples of knowledge, skills, and abilities.

- *Identify a relevant hypothesis based on a given investigation.*
- *Determine the strengths of a scientific investigation.*
- *Determine the weaknesses of a scientific investigation.*
- *Identify dependent, independent, and controlled variables.*
- *Determine whether a hypothesis is supported by evidence within a case study.*

Key terms

control variable. Something kept constant during an experiment.

dependent variable. What is measured in an experiment as a possible effect.

hypothesis. An educated guess that serves as a starting point for further testing.

independent variable. What is measured in an experiment as a possible cause.

variable. Something that changes.

Science is propelled by investigation. Scientists determine hypotheses based on known evidence and then create investigations to test the hypotheses. In order for information to be validated, scientists submit their ideas for scrutiny by other scientists. This process of investigation is important to society's understanding of the world. This TEAS task will focus on hypothesis and investigations.

Hypotheses are informed guesses about causal relationships that are generated by observation and initial data collection. In this way, they are not truly guesses about the outcome of an event. Scientists develop hypotheses only after they begin to have ideas about relationships. The hypothesis is a guiding idea to develop a strong investigation. During the investigation, the hypothesis will be accepted or rejected based on evidence.

Scientific investigations collect experimental data to develop theories. Scientists develop strategies in an investigation to control variables. Each experiment should manipulate only one variable: the independent variable (such as duration or concentration, plotted on the X–axis of a graph). All other variables should be kept the same in a controlled investigation. The dependent variable (such as growth or response, plotted on the Y–axis of a graph) is the observed condition that responds to the manipulation. This establishes a causal relationship between the independent and dependent variable.

Consider a scientist investigating the effectiveness of fertilizer on plant growth. She has 100 plants; 50 receive fertilizer and 50 do not. The independent variable is the fertilizer, and the dependent variable is the plant growth. All other variables, such as amount of sunlight, temperature, soil conditions, and type of plant, should be maintained the same (controlled) across all plants. It is important to review the methodology of any investigation to determine if it is valid. The TEAS will ask questions about investigations and variables.

After investigations, scientists analyze data to determine possible conclusions. The conclusions are based on evidence and subjected to scrutiny by other scientists. Scientists finally submit their evidence to journals, where the investigation and data are reviewed. Only the most reliable data should pass through this process. Scientists accept or reject hypotheses through this process.

S.3.4 Practice problems

Scientists believe that noise can affect the concentration of mice. They design an experiment to test this hypothesis. The scientists construct a maze and then have mice complete the maze. They test 500 mice. Half of the mice are required to run the maze with the same loud music playing in the background. The scientists then compare the time the mice took to complete the maze in silence vs. the loud music playing. It is found that mice complete the maze in half the time when it is quiet.

1. Which of the following is the dependent variable?

   A. Loud music playing

   B. Number of mice in the study

   C. Maze construction

   D. Time it takes to complete the maze

2. Which of the following statements is the hypothesis?

   A. Mice finish mazes faster when the environment is quiet.

   B. If there is loud noise, mice will complete the maze more slowly.

   C. Mazes are an effective way to test mice.

   D. Loud music makes mice finish mazes faster.

Mary and Ellen do a study for their science fair project. They measure height and stride length of several people on the tarmac in front of their school and come up with the following data.

Person #	Height (feet, inches)	Stride length (feet, inches)
1	5′	2′
2	5′6″	2′4″
3	6′	3′

3. For this experiment, identify the following.

   A. Dependent variable

   B. Independent variable

   C. Controlled conditions

   D. Possible hypothesis

Practice problem answers

S.3.1

1. Option C is correct. Kilometer is the most appropriate unit.
   - Liters measure volume, not distance.
   - Meters measure smaller lengths.
   - Centimeters measure much smaller lengths.
2. Option D is correct.
   - Option A is kilo.
   - Option B is hecta.
   - Option C is centi.
3. Option A is correct.
   - Volumetric pipettes measure volume.
   - Graduated cylinders measure volume
   - Rulers measure length.

S.3.2

1. Option B is correct.
   - Because the pills were taken all together, there is no way to know which pill is effective.
   - Although the data shows the blood pressure lowering for each client, no record is included of diet change or other lifestyle changes that lower blood pressure. The changes could be due to other factors.
   - Although the time is controlled, this is invalid without measuring the change in blood pressure at other times.
2. This is intentional bias. The researcher set up different practices for each client without accounting for the potential effect on outcome.
3. Option B is correct. The condition that is changed to measure its effect is the independent variable.
   - The term "data" refers to all the information gathered in the experiment.
   - Control refers to conditions that are kept consistent throughout an experiment.
   - Bias refers to a tendency of the experimenter to influence the results, knowingly or unknowingly, through their affective state.

S.3.3

1. Option B is correct.
   - Grams, milligrams, and micrograms are too small unit to measure that much weight.
2. Option A is correct.
   - Meters, centimeters, and micrometers are too small to be efficient in measuring the circumference of the Earth.
3. Option C is correct. Smoking causes deposition of tar in the lungs, making them less elastic. This is a primary cause of emphysema.
   - Overeating can cause temporary distress, but does not lead to severe respiratory problems.
   - Alcohol consumption causes intoxication, not respiratory problems.
   - Sleep deprivation causes tiredness, not respiratory problems.

S.3.4

1. Option D is correct.
   - The loud music is the independent variable.
   - Options B and C are variables, but they are controlled in the experiment.
2. Option B is correct.
   - Option A would be a conclusion statement after the data are analyzed.
   - Options C and D are not supported by the experimental data.
3. Dependent variable
   - Stride length

   Independent variable
   - Height

   Controlled conditions
   - Tarmac
   - Weather

   Possible hypothesis
   - Height affects stride length.
   - There is a positive correlation between height and stride length.

Science section quiz

1. Which of the following cavities is lined by the connective tissue peritoneum?
   A. Cephalic
   B. Thoracic
   C. Abdominal
   D. Pelvic

2. Which of the following is a hormone that mediates the fight-or-flight response?
   A. Insulin
   B. Glucagon
   C. Epinephrine
   D. Endorphin

3. Which of the following occurs if the epiglottis does not function properly?
   A. The client is unable to recall recent events.
   B. The client coughs because food goes into the trachea.
   C. The client cannot produce hormones from the pancreas.
   D. The client becomes reproductively sterile.

4. Which of the following composes the rings that support the trachea?
   A. Spongy bone
   B. Fibrous ligaments
   C. Elastic tendons
   D. Hyaline cartilage

5. Which of the following valves prevent backflow of blood from the arteries into the ventricle?
   A. Bicuspid
   B. Tricuspid
   C. Mitral
   D. Semilunar

6. Which of the following arteries supplies the heart with blood?
   A. Carotid
   B. Coronary
   C. Subclavian
   D. Brachiocephalic

7. Breakdown of which of the following begins in the small intestine?
   A. Fats
   B. Fiber
   C. Protein
   D. Carbohydrates

8. Which of the following are lymphatic capillaries that absorb fats?
   A. Lacteals
   B. Nodules
   C. Bronchioles
   D. Axons

9. Which of the following occurs to skeletal muscle as a result of acetylcholine released at the neuromuscular junction?
   A. Relaxation
   B. Peristalsis
   C. Contraction
   D. Eversion

10. Which of the following is the tube that carries both sperm and urine for release outside the body?
    A. Ureter
    B. Urethra
    C. Vas deferens
    D. Epididymis

11. Which of the following is the protein secreted by hair follicles in the integument?
    A. Collagen
    B. Fibrin
    C. Elastin
    D. Keratin

12. Which of the following is a portion of the brain that integrates nerve signals and hormonal secretions?
    A. Hypothalamus
    B. Adrenal gland
    C. Nucleus accumbens
    D. Medulla oblongata

13. Which of the following is the region of the kidney that contains the glomerulus of the nephron?
    A. Medulla
    B. Pelvis
    C. Cortex
    D. Adrenal

14. Which of the following antibody-secreting cells is triggered to proliferate upon vaccination?
    A. Erythrocytes
    B. B-lymphocytes
    C. Leukocytes
    D. T-lymphocytes

15. Which of the following bones supports the tongue and is the only bone in the body not anchored to other bones?
    A. Patella
    B. Coccyx
    C. Hyoid
    D. Scapula

16. Which of the following produces ammonia by deamination in the liver?
    A. Proteins
    B. Carbohydrates
    C. Nucleic acids
    D. Lipids

17. A cross between two heterozygous F1 plants produces a ratio of 15:1 in the F2 offspring. Which of the following best describes the ratio?
    A. Modified monohybrid ratio
    B. Modified dihybrid ratio
    C. Normal monohybrid ratio
    D. Normal dihybrid ratio

18. Which of the following is the smallest region in space where two electrons with opposite spins are paired?
    A. Shell
    B. Orbital
    C. Nucleus
    D. Period

19. Which of the following best describes matter in which the components cannot be broken down into simpler substances?
    A. Molecule
    B. Element
    C. Mixture
    D. Compound

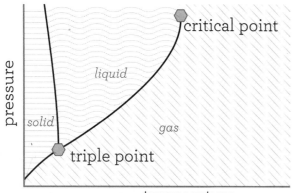

20. The graph shows the phases of water. Which of the following statements makes a correct prediction regarding phase change?
    A. Reducing pressure at a fixed temperature will generally convert a liquid to a solid.
    B. Solids have the highest temperature value at a given pressure.
    C. At the triple point, solids, liquids, and vapor forms disappear.
    D. At low temperatures and high pressures, solids are the only form present.

21. Which of the following reactions describes iron being reduced?
    A. $4Fe + 3O_2 \rightarrow 2Fe_2O_3$
    B. $Fe + O \rightarrow FeO$
    C. $3Fe_2O_3 + CO \rightarrow 2Fe_3O_4 + CO_2$
    D. $2Fe_2O_3 + 3H_2O \rightarrow Fe(OH)_3$

22. Which of the following formulas best summarizes a single replacement reaction?
    A. $A + B \rightarrow AB$
    B. $AB + C \rightarrow AC + B$
    C. $AB + CD \rightarrow AD + BC$
    D. $AB \rightarrow A + B$

23. A student measures 2,000 mL water into a cylinder. If water has a mass of 1 g/mL, which of the following is the approximate mass of the water?
    A. 200 mg
    B. 2 g
    C. 200 cg
    D. 20 hg

24. Offspring of parents who eat a diet low in omega-6 fatty acids have fewer health problems than offspring of parents who consume diets rich omega-6 fatty acids. Which of the following statements provides the most logical extension of this observation?
    A. The offspring of parents who were starved will be healthier than offspring of well-fed parents.
    B. Diets rich in omega-6 fatty acids are poor nutritional choices for long-term family health.
    C. Any high-calorie diet that omits omega-6 fatty acids is beneficial to long-term family health.
    D. Health outcomes of a person's diet are visible in the health of offspring rather than the individual.

When two closely related species of flour beetles, *T. confusum* and *T. castaneum*, were placed in a culture in equal numbers, *T. castaneum* increased in numbers while *T. confusum* experienced population decline. The growth difference in the changes of population most likely indicates that the energy consumption efficiency of *T. castaneum* is _____ *T. confusum*.

25. Which of the following correctly completes the sentence above?
    A. less than
    B. less variable than
    C. greater than
    D. more variable than

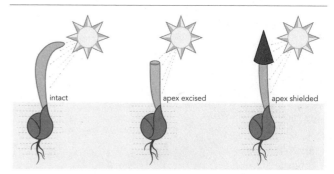

26. An investigation of the growth of a plant apex exposed to light as shown in the diagram was carried out under three conditions: intact apex, excised apex, and shielded apex. Which of the following conclusions is correct?
    A. Apex side exposed to light elongates slower than side away from light.
    B. Living cells that respond to light are exclusive to the shoot apex of plants.
    C. Plants will not respond to light even when the apex shield is removed.
    D. Tips exposed to light elongate evenly in response to light.

27. Which of the following muscle movements has synapses in the spinal cord rather than the brain?
   A. Reflex arc
   B. Contraction
   C. Relaxation
   D. Slow twitch

28. Which of the following structures is responsible for egg production?
   A. Vagina
   B. Fallopian tubes
   C. Ovaries
   D. Uterus

29. Which of the following integumentary structures produces sweat?
   A. Sudoriferous glands
   B. Sebaceous glands
   C. Ceruminous glands
   D. Mammary glands

30. Which of the following endocrine organs produces insulin?
   A. Thyroid
   B. Pituitary
   C. Adrenal gland
   D. Pancreas

31. Which of the following structures stores urine before excretion?
   A. Kidneys
   B. Ureters
   C. Bladder
   D. Urethra

32. Which of the following parts of the adult body makes white blood cells?
   A. Thymus
   B. Bone marrow
   C. Adenoid glands
   D. Liver

33. Which of the following structures is an irregularly shaped bone?
   A. Femur
   B. Metacarpal
   C. Rib
   D. Vertebra

34. The parathyroid is a component of which of the following organ systems?
   A. Lymphatic
   B. Nervous
   C. Endocrine
   D. Muscular

35. After passing through the stomach, food continues into which of the following digestive structures?
   A. Duodenum
   B. Jejunum
   C. Ileum
   D. Cecum

_____ are at a higher structural level of organization than _____.

36. Which of the following options completes the sentence?
   A. Organs; organ systems
   B. Cells; molecules
   C. Atoms; molecules
   D. Tissues; organs

37. In which of the following stages of embryological development are the main germ layers (ectoderm, endoderm, and mesoderm) formed?
   A. Blastula
   B. Morula
   C. Gastrula
   D. Fetus

38. Vaccinations are used to create which of the following types of immunity?
   A. Naturally acquired passive immunity
   B. Artificially acquired passive immunity
   C. Naturally acquired active immunity
   D. Artificially acquired active immunity

39. Which of the following nervous systems directs the skeletal muscles to respond in the body's fight-or-flight response?
   A. Enteric
   B. Central
   C. Parasympathetic
   D. Sympathetic

40. Which of the following tissues is responsible for contractions during peristalsis in the digestive tract?
   A. Smooth muscle
   B. Skeletal muscle
   C. Connective tissue
   D. Subcutaneous tissue

41. In which of the following organs are immune cells produced?
   A. Tonsils
   B. Spleen
   C. Lymph nodes
   D. Bone marrow

42. Exchange of gases occurs in which of the following structures of the respiratory system?
   A. Alveoli
   B. Bronchioles
   C. Trachea
   D. Pleura

43. Which of the following organelles gives rough endoplasmic reticulum its signature rough characteristic?
   A. Ribosomes
   B. Mitochondria
   C. Centrosomes
   D. Vacuoles

44. Which of the following is the number of different types of nucleotide bases found in DNA?
   A. 1
   B. 2
   C. 3
   D. 4

45. Which of the following measures volumes of liquids?
  A. Triple beam balance
  B. Meter stick
  C. Graduated cylinder
  D. Weigh boat

Soil samples

Nutrient	Sample 1	Sample 2
Nitrates	Yes	Yes
Phosphates	Yes	No

46. A student is testing the materials in two different soil samples. Which of the following assumptions can be inferred from the data presented in the table?
  A. Different soils contain different nutrients.
  B. Sample 1 is the best soil.
  C. Nitrates are more frequently found in soil than are phosphates.
  D. Most plants thrive in nitrate-rich soil.

47. A researcher wants to test the hypothesis that soy-based diets are superior to whole wheat-based diets for reproduction in a certain type of beetle. Which of the following describes how the researcher should best test this hypothesis?
  A. Record the number of eggs recovered from a single culture reared on soy vs. a single culture reared on whole wheat.
  B. Count the eggs recovered from 10 separate cultures reared on soy versus a single culture on whole wheat.
  C. Compare the eggs from 10 soy cultures versus 10 whole-wheat cultures.
  D. Record the eggs from one soy culture versus 10 whole-wheat cultures.

Science section quiz rationales

1. Option C is correct. The abdominal cavity is lined by peritoneum. Cephalic refers to the head. Thoracic refers to the chest. Pelvic refers to the hip area. See S.1.1 for related information.

2. Option C is correct. Epinephrine mediates the fight-or-flight response. Insulin and glucagon are involved in glucose homeostasis. Endorphins are the body's natural painkillers. See S.1.1 for related information.

3. Option B is correct. The epiglottis shuts the larynx to prevent food being aspirated into the trachea. The epiglottis is not part of the brain or reproductive system. Pancreatic hormones are produced from the islets of Langerhans. See S.1.2 for related information.

4. Option D is correct. Tracheal rings are made of hyaline cartilage. Ligaments connect bone to bone. Tendons connect muscle to bone. See S.1.2 for related information.

5. Option D is correct. Semilunar valves, which are present in both aorta and pulmonary arteries, prevent blood backflow. The bicuspid, or mitral, valve is located between the left atrium and ventricle. The tricuspid valve is located between the right atrium and ventricle. See S.1.3 for related information.

6. Option B is correct. Coronary arteries bring oxygenated blood to the heart. Carotid arteries take blood to the brain. Subclavian arteries supply the right and left side of the body. The brachiocephalic artery divides into the right common carotid and right subclavian arteries. See S.1.3 for related information.

7. Option A is correct. Breakdown of fats begins in the small intestine. Fiber is not digestible. Breakdown of protein begins in the stomach. Breakdown of carbohydrates begins in the mouth. See S.1.4 for related information.

8. Option A is correct. Lacteals are lymphatic branches that absorb dietary fats. Lymph nodes do not absorb fats. Bronchioles are tubes that carry air into and out of lungs. Axons are extensions of nerves that participate in signal transduction. See S.1.4 for related information.

9. Option C is correct. Acetylcholine is involved in skeletal muscle contraction. Peristalsis is the movement of food through the intestine. Eversion (turning something inside-out) does not occur in muscle. See S.1.5 for related information.

10. Option B is correct. The urethra carries both sperm and urine out of the body. The ureter carries urine from the kidneys to the bladder. The vas deferens takes sperm from the testes to the urethra. The epididymis takes sperm from the seminiferous tubules to the vas deferens. See S.1.6 for related information.

11. Option D is correct. Hair follicles produce hair, which is made of keratin. See S.1.7 for related information.

12. Option A is correct. The hypothalamus integrates neural signals and endocrine secretions and releases releasing hormones that act on the pituitary gland. The adrenal gland produces several hormones, but does not integrate nerve signals and does not serve as a master regulatory endocrine gland. The nucleus accumbens is not part of the endocrine system. The medulla oblongata is part of the brainstem, not an endocrine organ. See S.1.8 for related information.

13. Option C is correct. The glomerulus and proximal and distal convoluted tubules are located in the cortex. Henle's loop descends into the medulla. The pelvis is the area of the kidney where the collecting tubules discharge urine for transport to the bladder through the ureter. The adrenal glands sit atop the kidneys but do not contain nephrons. See S.1.9 for related information.

14. Option B is correct. B-lymphocytes make antibodies and proliferate on vaccination. Erythrocytes are red blood cells, which do not proliferate upon vaccination. Leukocytes, or white blood cells, do not proliferate upon vaccination. T-lymphocytes do not secrete antibodies and do not typically proliferate upon vaccination. See S.1.10 for related information.

15. Option C is correct. The hyoid bone supports the tongue and is not attached to other bones. The patella is found in the knee and is articulated to the tibia, fibula, and femur. The coccyx is the tail bone and is attached to the rest of the spine. The scapula is the bone of the shoulder and is attached to the clavicle and humerus. See S.1.11 for related information.

16. Option A is correct. The liver deaminates amino acids to produce ammonia, which is then converted to urea. Carbohydrates and lipids do not have an amino group. Nucleic acids contain amino groups, but are not a major source of ammonia. See S.2.1 for related information.

17. Option B is correct. The normal dihybrid ratio is 9:3:3:1, so this is a modified dihybrid ratio. The monohybrid ratio is 3:1. See S.2.3 for related information.

18. Option B is correct. An orbital contains paired electrons with opposite spins. A shell is an energy level usually containing many electrons. A nucleus contains protons and neutrons, not electrons. A period refers to the energy shells of an electron. See S.2.4 for related information.

19. Option B is correct. An element is a substance made of a single type of atoms that are generally held together by physical forces. A molecule contains atoms that have been chemically combined. A mixture contains substances mixed together physically in varying proportions. A compound is a molecule made by chemical reaction between atoms. See S.2.5 for related information.

20. Option D is correct. The graph shows that at low temperatures and high pressures, only solids are present. The graph also shows that reducing pressure on the Y-axis at a fixed value on the X-axis will more likely convert a liquid to a vapor. Liquid and vapor generally have higher temperatures at a given pressure. At the triple point, solids, liquids, and vapor coexist. See S.2.6 for related information.

21. Option C is correct. In this reaction, iron (III) oxide is losing oxygen to CO, and iron is going from Fe(III) to Fe(II). Therefore, iron is reduced. When oxygen is added in Option A, Fe is oxidized, not reduced. In this reaction, Fe is transferring electrons to oxygen and going from Fe(0) to Fe(III) oxidation state. In Option B, oxygen is added, and iron is going from Fe(0) to Fe(II) oxidation state. In Option D, water is added to iron (III) oxide, and iron does not change oxidation state. See S.2.7 for related information.

22. Option B is correct. This is a single replacement reaction because element B is replaced by element C. Options A and D are synthesis reactions. Option C is a double replacement reaction. See S.2.7 for related information.

23. Option D is correct. Twenty hectograms is the same as 2 kg, which is the mass of water measured. Option A is the mass of 0.2 mL water. Option B is the mass of 2 mL water. Option C the mass of 20 mL water. See S.3.1 for related information.

24. Option B is correct. The stem identifies omega-6 fatty acids as being problematical in the long term, so this statement is correct. Starvation is a serious nutritional issue. It is unlikely that parental starvation benefits offspring more than the parents being well-fed. While omega-6 is a poor nutritional choice, it doesn't follow that any diet high in calories is likely to benefit health. Although dietary choices can affect offspring later, it is very likely that the diet also influences the individual consuming it. See S.3.2 for related information.

25. Option C is correct. Energy consumption is necessary for growth in all animals. Therefore, population growth is positively correlated with the consumption of food (i.e., energy). See S.3.3 for related information.

26. Option A is correct. This causes the plant apex to bend toward light. Although the experiment reveals that the apex is necessary for the light response, it doesn't mean other living cells do not. Leaves also respond to light. There is no indication that the apex shield permanently affects apex function. This was not part of the described experiment. Apexes exposed to light elongate unevenly, causing bending. See S.3.4 for related information.

27. Option A is correct. A reflex is an involuntary reaction to stimulus. Contraction is a movement of muscle that pulls protein tighter together. Relaxation is a movement of muscle that allows protein to stretch. Slow twitch is a type of muscle metabolism that provides endurance for the muscle. See S.1.5 for related information.

28. Option C is correct. Ovaries are the sites of egg production. The vagina is the tube that leads to the uterus. Fallopian tubes carry eggs to the uterus, where a fertilized egg grows into a fetus. See S.1.6 for related information.

29. Option A is correct. Sudoriferous glands produce sweat and come in two varieties: eccrine and apocrine glands. Sebaceous glands produce oily secretions. Ceruminous glands produce wax. Mammary glands produce milk. See S.1.7 for related information.

30. Option D is correct. The pancreas produces insulin. The thyroid gland produces thyroid hormone. The pituitary releases hormones that control other glands in the body. Adrenal glands produce steroids that control metabolism, flight-or-fight response, and stress regulation. See S.1.8 for related information.

31. Option C is correct. The bladder stores urine. Kidneys filter blood and make urine. Ureters carry urine from the kidneys to the bladder. The urethra connects the bladder to the exterior of the body. See S.1.9 for related information.

32. Option B is correct. Bone marrow is where many cells of the blood are made, including white blood cells. The thymus holds T-cells until they mature. Prevent infection by trapping germs that have been inhaled. The liver produces globulin that can aid the immune system. See S.1.10 for related information.

33. Option D is correct. Vertebrae are irregular bones. The femur is a long bone. Metacarpals are short bones. Ribs are flat bones. See S.1.11 for related information.

34. Option C is correct. The pancreas is a component of the endocrine system, and it produces several important hormones, including insulin. See S.1.8 for related information.

35. Option A is correct. After passing through the stomach, food continues into the duodenum. The jejunum is part of the small intestine located between the duodenum and ileum. The ileum is part of the small intestine located between the jejunum and the cecum. The cecum is a pouch that serves as the junction between the small and large intestines. See S.1.4 for related information.

36. Option B is correct. Cells are at a higher level of organization than molecules. Organ systems are at a higher level of organization than organs. Molecules are at a higher level of organization than atoms. Organs are at a higher level of organization than tissues. See S.1.1 for related information.

37. Option C is correct. During the gastrula stage, the germ layers are formed. During the blastula stage, the inner cell mass and blastopore are formed. Embryogenesis is completed by the fetus stage. See S.1.1 for related information.

38. Option D is correct. A vaccine is deliberately introduced to the host, so it is not considered naturally acquired. The immunity is considered active because the host is responding to the antigen. See S.1.10 for related information.

39. Option D is correct. The sympathetic nervous system activates the body's fight-or-flight response. In the presence of stress, the heart beats faster and stronger, more blood is carried to the vital organs, and the pupils dilate to prepare the body to defend itself. The enteric peripheral nervous system controls the digestive glands. The central nervous system typically produces reflex arcs and processes external stimuli. The parasympathetic nervous system promotes responses that are the opposite of the sympathetic system, such as digestion and maintenance. See S.1.5 for related information.

40. Option A is correct. The lining of the hollow organs of the digestive system, such as the esophagus, stomach, and intestines, is comprised of smooth muscle tissue, which creates the peristalsis needed to push undigested food through the body. See S.1.4 for related information.

41. Option D is correct. Immune cells are produced in the body's bone marrow. Immune cells mature and get activated in the tonsils, spleen, and lymph nodes. See S.1.10 for related information.

42. Option A is correct. The alveoli are the structures in the respiratory system in which the exchange of gases occurs. Although the bronchioles, trachea, and pleura are components of the respiratory system, they are not directly responsible for gas exchange. See S.1.2 for related information.

43. Option A is correct. Ribosomes on the surface of the endoplasmic reticulum (ER) give it a rough characteristic, as opposed to smooth ER, which lacks ribosomes. Mitochondria are energy-producing organelles that are independent of ER. Centrosomes are involved in cell division and not part of the ER. Vacuoles are sacs of fluids in the cytoplasm arising from the Golgi apparatus or cell membrane and are not part of the ER. See S.1.1 for related information.

44. Option D is correct. There are four nucleotide bases in DNA. There is one type of sugar in DNA. There are two strands of DNA in a double helix. Three nucleic acids make a codon. See S.2.2 for related information.

45. Option C is correct. Graduated cylinders measure volume of liquids. Balances measure mass. Meter sticks measure length. Weigh boats are used to protect scales. See S.3.1 for related information.

46. Option A is correct. Because Sample 1 contains phosphates and Sample 2 does not, you can conclude that different soils contain different nutrients. See S.3.2 for related information.

47. Option C is correct. The protocol in this option gives enough replications on each diet to determine the accuracy and precision of the experiment and increase the statistical significance of the data. See S.3.4 for related information.

English and language usage

The objectives for the English and language usage section of the TEAS are organized in three categories.

Conventions of standard English (E.1)   *9 questions*

E.1.1. Use conventions of standard English spelling.
E.1.2. Use conventions of standard English punctuation.
E.1.3. Analyze various sentence structures.

Knowledge of language (E.2)   *9 questions*

E.2.1. Use grammar to enhance clarity in writing.
E.2.2. Distinguish between formal and informal language.
E.2.3. Apply basic knowledge of the elements of the writing process.
E.2.4. Develop a well-organized paragraph.

Vocabulary acquisition (E.3)   *6 questions*

E.3.1. Use context clues to determine the meaning of words or phrases.
E.3.2. Determine the meaning of words by analyzing word parts.

Remember, there are 24 scored English and Language Usage items on the TEAS. These are divided as shown above. In addition, there will be four unscored pretest items that can be in any of these categories.

E.1.1 *Use conventions of standard English spelling.*

What's the difference between "aural" and "oral"? Not much if you're speaking them aloud, but it's a pretty big one if you're reading a prescription to determine whether to administer a medication in the ear (aural) or the mouth (oral). Identifying homophones like this is just one of the conventions of spelling that is essential to reading and writing accurately. For this task, you'll need to know common spelling rules, such as those for forming plurals, and the exceptions to those rules. You'll need to be able to identify incorrectly spelled words and determine the correct selection of homophones based on context. Be sure to master the most common spelling rules and to browse online resources for spelling.

We've all probably heard the mnemonic *I before E except after C or when sounding like A as in neighbor and weigh.* There are many more spelling rules that you could learn, but it's best to master the most common ones and to know some common exceptions to those rules. Here are some rules you should certainly know for the TEAS.

I before E: This rule is well known, but it has plenty of exceptions. Examples include the following.

I before E	Except after C	Sounding like A	Exceptions
achieve	conceive	their	caffeine
belief	deceive	reign	neither
chief	perceive	vein	weird

Drop the final E: When adding a suffix to a root that ends in E, drop the E if the suffix begins with a vowel but not before a suffix beginning with a consonant.

Suffix beginning with a vowel	Suffix beginning with a consonant	Exceptions
guide + ance = guidance	derange + ment = derangement	due + ly = duly
hide + ing = hiding	like + ly = likely	peace + able = peaceable
titrate + ing = titrating	like + ness = likeness	true + ly = truly

Double the final consonant: When adding a suffix to a root that ends in a single consonant, double the consonant if a single vowel precedes the consonant and the consonant ends an accented syllable or one-syllable word. In some cases, though, there isn't a definitive spelling for a word when it comes to this rule.

Conditions met	Conditions not met	On the fence
admit + ed = admitted	loop + ing = looping	travel + ing = traveling, travelling
bat + ed = batted	light + ed = lighted	cancel +ed = canceled, cancelled
stop + ing = stopping	visit + ed = visited	

This objective includes, but is not limited to, the following examples of knowledge, skills, and abilities.

- *Spell words using common rules for English spelling (e.g., I before E, dropping the final E, changing the final Y to I, doubling a final consonant).*

- *Identify common words that are exceptions to common rules for English spelling (e.g., receive, vein, height, protein, neither).*

- *Identify plural forms of common words found in the English language.*

- *Reference in-text examples for self-correction of spelling errors.*

- *Know homophones and homographs (e.g., their/ they're, its/it's).*

ENGLISH

Change the final Y to I: When adding a suffix to a root ending in Y preceded by a consonant, change the Y to I unless the suffix begins with I.

Conditions met	Vowel before Y	Suffix begins with I	Exceptions
beauty + ful = beautiful	annoy + ance = annoyance	apply + ing = applying	memory + ize = memorize
merry + ment = merriment	lay + ing = laying	decay + ing = decaying	day + ly = daily
pacify + ed = pacified	stay + ed = stayed	spy + ing = spying	

You should also be well-versed in the rules for making plurals. Here are some things to keep in mind.

- For regular plurals, you only need to add -s. Examples: apple/apples, car/cars, nurse/nurses.

- Add -es for words ending in -ch, -s, -sh, -x, or -z. Examples: dash/dashes, lunch/lunches, boss/bosses.

- Change to -ves for some words ending in -f or -fe. Examples: elf/elves, life/lives, self/selves. Exceptions: chief/chiefs, proof/proofs.

In addition, you'll need to be able to use context to identify homophones, or words that are pronounced the same but are spelled differently, and homographs, which are words that are spelled the same but have different meanings. Here is just a small set of examples.

Key terms

homograph. Words spelled the same but that have different meanings.

homophone. Words pronounced the same but that have different meanings.

mnemonic. A pattern or other device to help remember something.

plural. More than one.

Homophones	Homographs
ate/eight	bat – a piece of sporting equipment/a winged animal
bare/bear	bow – to bend at the waist/a pair of tied loops
hole/whole	content – happy/all that is contained within something
its/it's	digest – a condensed version of a text/to process food
seam/seem	minute – 60 seconds of time/very small

E.1.1 Practice problems

The billionaire had a compound in the desert, the shear size of which made it seam like a whole other country.

1. Which of the following correctly describes an error in the sentence above?

   A. The homograph "desert" should be "dessert."

   B. The homophone "shear" should be "sheer."

   C. The homograph "seam" should be "seem."

   D. The homophone "whole" should be "hole."

He found it inconceivable that his partner had leapt to the wrong conclusion regarding the capital they had alloted to the project.

2. Which of the following words is misspelled in the sentence above?

   A. inconceivable

   B. leapt

   C. capital

   D. alloted

3. Perform a search and make a list of 10 homophones and 10 homographs that you didn't previously know. Write out definitions for each word.

E.1.2 Use conventions of standard English punctuation.

Punctuation is like a system of road signs for written language.
It provides direction as you journey through a piece of writing, and mastery of punctuation allows you to read and write with clarity. To successfully answer questions for this task, you'll need to study the rules for using commas, periods, question marks, colons, semicolons, apostrophes, quotation marks, and more. There are many great websites to reference for rules on using punctuation, but be sure to distinguish between established punctuation rules and matters of opinion.

One of the most important concepts that guide the use of punctuation is its use in clarifying various types of sentences—simple, compound, and complex. An example is the use of a comma prior to the conjunction in a compound sentence (i.e., one with two independent clauses).

> I studied assiduously for my punctuation test,
> and my score reflected my hard work.

The comma in this sentence indicates that what follows will be a second independent clause rather than another object of the preposition "for." Commas, along with colons and semicolons, help us identify independent and dependent clauses, and interpret how they interact to build compound and complex sentences, which are covered in more detail in the next section.

The comma is used for a multitude of purposes, from dividing items in a series to indicating pauses in the flow of a sentence. Understanding the rules governing commas is critical to succeeding on this task of the TEAS exam. You'll need to be careful to distinguish between rules and preferences. For example, the serial comma, also known as the Oxford comma, is the comma before the "and" in a simple series of items. It is preferred in many forms of writing but not all. Questions on the TEAS address rules, not preferences, so the omission of a serial comma would not be considered an error. Using a comma without a conjunction to separate two independent clauses, however, is the kind of error that you will need to recognize on the TEAS.

You'll also need to recognize how to use quotation marks, apostrophes, end marks, and other punctuation. This sentence provides just a taste of how these can interact.

> "It's not easy to write well," she declared. "At least,
> not if that guy's memoir is any indication!"

This example demonstrates a number of concepts.

- Quotation marks are used for direct quotations, and a comma is used before the closed quote if there is additional text in the sentence.

- An apostrophe is used for conjunctions and to indicate possession.

- An exclamation mark is used to indicate both the end of the sentence and strong feeling or high volume.

Any concrete rule regarding punctuation is fair game for this task on the TEAS, so be sure to brush up using a variety of sources.

This objective includes, but is not limited to, the following examples of knowledge, skills, and abilities.

- *Demonstrate knowledge of sentence punctuation patterns (e.g., simple, compound, complex).*

- *Use a comma to clarify meaning (e.g., placement in compound sentences, after introductory elements, with dependent phrases and clauses, around nonessential elements, in a series, with adjectives).*

- *Use direct and indirect quotations following standard English rules.*

- *Use end marks to clarify meaning.*

Key terms

apostrophe. Punctuation mark that denotes omission of letters and possessive case.

colon. Punctuation mark used in introduction of a quote or list, ratio, and time.

comma. Punctuation mark used to separate parts of sentences.

end marks. Punctuation marks that end sentences: period, question mark, and exclamation mark.

exclamation mark. End mark that denotes strong feeling.

parentheses. Punctuation marks that set off explanatory material within text.

period. End mark that denotes the end of a standard sentence.

question mark. End mark that denotes a query.

quotation marks. Punctuation marks that denote spoken or other quoted text.

ENGLISH

E.1.2 Practice problems

1. Which of the following examples is a correctly punctuated compound sentence?

   A. I've been running all over town; but now it's time for me to relax.

   B. I plan on taking it easy for the rest of the day and no one has any cause to bother me.

   C. Perhaps I'll see if the spa is open, and if my favorite masseuse is available.

   D. Getting a massage would be fantastically relaxing, and I feel that I've earned it today.

2. Which of the following examples is a correct method for punctuating this quotation?

   A. "The key to wisdom," she said. "Is recognizing that the breadth of one's knowledge is never as great as the gulf of one's ignorance."

   B. "The key to wisdom," she said, "is recognizing that the breadth of one's knowledge is never as great as the gulf of one's ignorance."

   C. "The key to wisdom is recognizing that the breadth of one's knowledge is never as great as the gulf of one's ignorance." she said.

   D. "The key to wisdom is recognizing that the breadth of one's knowledge is never as great as the gulf of one's ignorance," She said.

3. Conduct your own research and make a list of rules for the use of commas. Be sure to include only rules, not instances of preferred usage.

E.1.3 *Analyze various sentence structures.*

We all know what a sentence is. Simply put, it is a set of words combined to express a complete thought. If only it were that easy! For this TEAS task, you'll need to be familiar with the complexities of sentence structure, including types of sentences and how they are built using sentence parts, including subjects, predicates, phrases, and clauses. You'll also need to know the parts of speech and how they are combined within a sentence. Mastering the definitions for all the glossary items listed in this chapter will be critical for success at this task. It would be a good idea to practice diagramming a range of sentences.

Parts of speech refer to how words are used in sentences. There are generally considered to be eight parts of speech: nouns, pronouns, verbs, adjectives, adverbs, prepositions, conjunctions, and interjections. Some grammar experts consider articles (a, an, the) as parts of speech in place of interjections. These parts of speech combine in various ways to make up sentence parts, including the subject and predicate that make up any given sentence. The simple subject is the noun (or noun substitute), and the complete subject includes the noun and all its complements and modifiers. The simple predicate is the verb, and the complete predicate includes the verb and all its complements and modifiers. Take this example:

> The cute, furry dog wagged its tail with joy.

The simple subject is the noun "dog," and the complete subject includes the article and modifiers: "The cute, furry dog". The simple predicate is the verb "wagged," and the complete predicate includes the direct object ("its tail") and the prepositional modifier ("with joy").

Clauses and phrases are also constructions that you should be able to recognize. A clause is a group of words that contains a subject and a verb. An independent clause is basically a simple sentence and can stand on its own. A dependent clause cannot stand on its own because it doesn't finish a complete thought. A phrase is a group of words that doesn't have a subject and a verb, and it is used as a single part of speech. Consider the following examples.

> Independent clause: I am hungry.

> Dependent clause: Although I've been snacking all day...

> Phrase: ...for sweets

These can be combined to make a complex sentence.

> Although I've been snacking all day, I am hungry for sweets.

A good way to enhance your understanding of sentence construction and the parts of speech is to practice diagramming sentences. There are plenty of online resources available with information on diagramming sentences and opportunities for practice. Here's just one example of how to diagram a sentence.

> The brawny lumberjack swung his ax with awful force.

The subject, verb, and object are all on the top line, separated by vertical lines. Their modifiers extend below them. In the case of the prepositional phrase, the preposition extends from the word it modifies and then introduces the prepositional object with its modifiers.

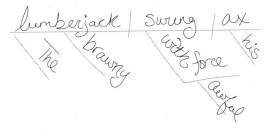

This objective includes, but is not limited to, the following examples of knowledge, skills, and abilities.

- *Identify patterns of simple, compound, complex, and compound-complex sentences.*

- *Combine dependent and independent clauses.*

- *Use the "Eight Parts of Speech": noun, pronoun, verb, adjective, adverb, preposition, conjunction, interjection.*

- *Use sentence parts (e.g., subject, predicate, object, indirect object, complement) to create coherent sentence structures.*

Key terms

adjective. Word or phrase that describes or modifies a noun.

adverb. Word or phrase that describes or modifies an adjective, verb, or other adverb.

article. Words (a and an) that refer to nouns.

complement. Sentence part that gives more information about a subject or object.

conjunction. A connecting word.

dependent clause. A group of words that includes a subject and verb but cannot stand alone as a complete sentence.

independent clause. A group of words that includes a subject and predicate and can stand alone as a complete sentence.

indirect object. The person or thing to whom or which something is done.

interjection. Words or phrases that represent short bursts of emotion.

modifier. A word or group of words that provides description for another word.

noun. A person, place, thing, or idea.

object. A word or group of words that receives the action of a verb.

phrase. A group of words that work together as a unit.

predicate. The part of a sentence that explains what the subject does or is like.

preposition. A word that describes relationships between other words.

pronoun. A word that takes the place of a noun.

subject. The main noun of a sentence that is doing or being.

verb. A word that describes an action or state of being.

ENGLISH

E.1.3 Practice problems

1. Which of the following examples is a compound-complex sentence?

   A. The large, sandy beach was packed with people, and they had all come for one reason.

   B. Although they didn't realize it at the time, this would prove to be a day they would never forget.

   C. Just as the concert started, the crowd looked to the sky, and the clouds parted.

   D. The sun came out and was surrounded by a rainbow halo that brought gasps of awe from the concert-goers.

2. Optimizing the time you spend enjoying life is the key to happiness.
   Which of the following is the simple subject in the sentence above?

   A. Optimizing

   B. time

   C. you

   D. life

3. Diagram the following sentences:

   The pool in my neighborhood is always packed with kids.

   The boy and the girl played catch for hours.

   He ran really fast, but the bus left without him.

Practice problem answers

E.1.1

1. Option B is correct. The words "desert" and "dessert" are actually homophones, and "desert" is properly used in the sentence, meaning a hot, arid region. The word "shear" means to cut the hair from, and "sheer" in this context would mean unqualified. While "seam" should be "seem" in the sentence, this is not a homograph but a homophone. The use of "whole," meaning "entire," is correct for this sentence.

2. Option D is correct. The spelling of this word should follow the "double the final consonant" rule: allotted.
   - Option A is spelled correctly. It follows the "I before E except after C" rule.
   - Option B is the correct spelling for the past tense of "leap".
   - Option C is the correct spelling for the homophone that refers to accumulated money.

E.1.2

1. Option D is correct. This sentence includes two independent clauses, and it is correctly punctuated by including a comma before the conjunction.
   - A comma, not a semicolon, should be used before a conjunction separating two independent clauses.
   - Option B has two independent clauses, so a comma should be used before the conjunction that separates the clauses.
   - Option C is not a compound sentence because there is only one subject (I). The comma before the "and" should not be included.

2. Option B is correct. This quotation is correctly punctuated by including a comma before the end quotation mark that leads to non-quotation text and another comma before beginning the quotation again.
   - By including the period in the non-quotation portion of this text, the writer has divided the quotation into two fragments. This is incorrect.
   - Using a period before an end quotation mark that is followed by additional text for the same sentence is incorrect.
   - Capitalizing the first word after a quotation (she) is incorrect if that word is part of the same sentence.

3. Rules that you could have listed include the following.
   - Commas are used to separate items in a series.
   - When a degree or certification is included after a person's name, it should be set off with commas.
   - When directly addressing a person, the person's name or title should be set off with commas.
   - When dates include the day of the month and the year, a comma should be included before the year.
   - Commas are used to separate geographic elements, such as between cities and their states.
   - An example of preferred usage that should not be included among rules would be the serial, or Oxford, comma. This is the comma before the "and" in a series of items.

E.1.3

1. Option C is correct. This is a compound-complex sentence that includes two independent and one dependent clause.
   - Option A is a compound sentence. There is no dependent clause, so it is not complex. There is just one independent clause, so it is not compound.
   - Option B is a complex sentence. There is just one independent clause, so it is not compound.
   - Option D is a simple sentence with a compound verb and four phrases.

2. Option A is correct. This subject is what's referred to as a gerund, or a verb that takes the form of a noun. It is the "who" or "what" that is the subject of the predicate "is."
   - The word "time" modifies the subject of the sentence.
   - The word "you" modifies the word "time."
   - The word "life" is the object of the phrase "enjoying life."

3.

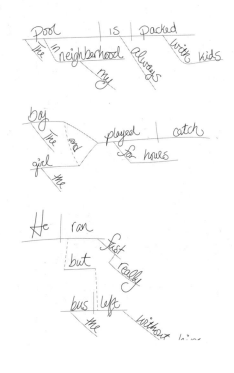

E.2.1 *Use grammar to enhance clarity in writing.*

Clarity in communication requires a common understanding between the writer and the reader. This is where grammar comes in. Grammar is the set of conventions that provide commonly accepted ways to demonstrate relationships and convey meaning in language. This TEAS task requires you to recognize both good and poor use of grammar, as well as precise versus ambiguous language. To prepare for this task, take note of reading passages you encounter that are unclear. Ask yourself why the passage is unclear and how it could be made clearer. How does the passage deviate from good grammar and good word choice, and how would you fix it?

Prescriptive grammar is an approach to language focused on establishing norms of correct and incorrect usage. Since the TEAS focuses on a concrete assessment of your knowledge, questions for this task focus on understanding the grammar rules that provide clarity in writing. You'll be asked to make judgments based on reading passages, but those judgments should be based on commonly accepted understandings rather than preference or opinion.

Perhaps the most fundamental element in grammar is the complete sentence. Sentence structure was addressed in detail in task E.1.3. For this task, you'll need to be able to recognize complete sentences, fragments, and run-on sentences. For example:

> Beat it! – A complete sentence with the understood subject "you"

> Depending on how you say it. – A fragment because the thought is not complete

> He really is a good guy he just sometimes loses his patience. – A run-on sentence due to the lack of a conjunction or appropriate punctuation

Transition words, including the conjunctions that would fix the run-on above, are essential in connecting ideas and clarifying the relationship between those ideas. You should be able to identify appropriate transition words based on context and recognize when a transition word is misused or another word is needed for clarity. This table provides examples of the types of transitions and specific transition words and phrases.

Transition type	Examples
Agreement	also, likewise, in addition, similarly
Opposition	but, although, then again, conversely
Cause	if, unless, in order to, in the event that
Examples	like, including, in other words, for example
Effect	therefore, consequently, accordingly, as a result
Conclusion	after all, in short, altogether, ultimately
Chronology	before, after, in the meantime, suddenly
Location	here, there, wherever, adjacent to

This objective includes, but is not limited to, the following examples of knowledge, skills, and abilities.

- *Recognize complete sentences.*

- *Use transition words (e.g., but, and, next, however, therefore) to clarify relationships.*

- *Be aware of past, present, and future tense.*

- *Choose precise diction (e.g., annoyed or angry or furious).*

- *Identify and eliminate ambiguous language (e.g., "and stuff").*

Key terms

diction. The style of writing determined by word choice.

fragment. An incomplete sentence.

perfective. A verb for an item that has been completed.

prescriptive grammar. Specific rules for using language and grammar.

progressive. A verb that shows something is currently happening.

run-on sentence. A sentence with extra parts not joined properly.

tense. Past, present, and future times.

transition word. Words that link or introduce ideas.

subject-verb agreement. Matching like numbers of subjects and verbs: singular with singular, plural with plural.

pronoun-antecedent agreement. Matching like numbers of pronouns and their antecedents: singular with singular, plural with plural.

ENGLISH

Tense, which is usually demonstrated by forms of verbs, is another way that we express a reference to time. The basic tenses are past, present, and future, but tense can also capture the aspect of an action. The aspect is either progressive, meaning incomplete, or perfective, meaning complete.

		Time		
		PAST	PRESENT	FUTURE
	NONE/SIMPLE	wrote	writes	will write
Aspect	PROGRESSIVE	was writing	is writing	will be writing
	PERFECTIVE	had written	has written	will have written

You'll need to be able to recognize when tenses are misused or don't agree within a given writing passage.

Word choice, or diction, is also foundational to clear communication. You'll need to be able to identify which choices are best for a given context. For example, the words "friendly," "courteous," and "lovely" all could be listed as synonyms for "nice." But would all of these really be an appropriate replacement for "nice" in the following sentence?

> She loved taking long walks in the sun on nice days like this.

There are a number of other grammar conventions that you'll need to apply, such as subject-verb agreement and pronoun-antecedent agreement. For this task, any grammar rule is fair game, so be sure to review a number of good grammar resources.

E.2.1 Practice problems

His daughter was an intrepid traveler, and no amount of coaxing is going to keep her from taking that cruise to Antarctica.

1. Which of the following describes the grammar problem in the sentence above?

   A. Inappropriate transition word choice

   B. Tense disagreement

   C. Poor diction

   D. Ambiguous word choice

He was thoroughly disappointed in his performance, _____ he pledged to redouble his efforts in his training regimen.

2. Which of the following transition words/phrases is most appropriate to complete the sentence?

   A. although

   B. in other words

   C. accordingly

   D. meanwhile

3. Practice your diction by reading a passage from your favorite book or a magazine article that appeals to you. Evaluate the author's word choice and brainstorm replacements for a number of the words in the passage. Do the replacement words enhance the clarity? Do they detract from it? What in the context helps you determine the best word choice?

E.2.2 *Distinguish between formal and informal language.*

Like chameleons changing their colors to match their environment, good writers should match their language to suit the intended audience. For example, slang, colloquialisms, and "loaded" language containing value judgments would be out of place in a research paper. As a reader, you should be able to identify the correct language for the setting. For this task, you need to evaluate language and match it to the correct audience.

Certain modes of writing—research papers, business communication, journalism—have conventions beyond simple good grammar. The audience for these modes of communication has common understandings and expectations that the writer must understand. For instance, a scientific paper should use neutral language in reporting data because an objective approach is expected. Some business acronyms (EOD, ROI) can be used without explanation in business communication. Journalistic reporting is expected to address the "who, what, why, when, and where" efficiently. While these conventions morph with the times, you should be able to identify the tone and key words that will tip you to the intended audience for a given piece of writing. Formal genres you should be able to identify include business letters, speeches, textbook articles, science reports, news stories, and essays.

Informal writing has its place, too. You wouldn't expect a text message from your friend to begin with "To whom it may concern." Narratives often benefit from informal language to create a feeling of realism or to set a tone. Slang and colloquialisms can provide otherwise unstated information about the time and place in which the communication originated. Take the following examples.

Decade	Slang	Meaning
1920s	All wet	erroneous idea or individual
	Bee's knees	extraordinary person, place, or thing
	Clam	a dollar
1950s	Cat	a hip person
	Dig	understand
	Gig	a job
1970s	Far out	cool
	Skinny	the truth or real story
	Psych	you've been tricked

Sure, some of these are still used today, but they can help to create an atmosphere that captures a day and age. Using colloquialisms can make a piece of writing feel more conversational and intimate, a style that can be beneficial in informal communication. You'll need to be able to recognize instances of slang and colloquialisms in writing passages for this task of the TEAS. Also, recognize when an author is using the second person (addressing the reader as "you"). This is a good indication that the piece is informal.

This objective includes, but is not limited to, the following examples of knowledge, skills, and abilities.

- *Given several short passages, choose which language fits a scenario.*
- *Identify language that is formal (e.g., academic, professional, public setting).*
- *Identify language that is informal (e.g., slang, colloquialisms).*
- *Be able to identify the narrator's setting/situation from given information (e.g., information provided in audio or in text format).*

Key terms

colloquialism. An informal word or phrase.

informal. A relaxed, unofficial style.

formal. A style that follows conventional rules.

second person. A narrative mode that addresses the reader as "you."

slang. Informal language usually tied to a specific group of people.

For questions on this task, you'll most likely need to evaluate the language in one or more passages and determine the appropriate scenario. Look for key words and phrases that can help identify the setting or the intended audience. When you're reading these passages, ask yourself the following questions.

- Is the author using conventions that seem specific to a certain type of audience?

- Does the author use slang or colloquialism?

- Is the language neutral or does it imply value judgments?

- What kind of descriptors does the author use and do they color the reader's interpretation of the material?

E.2.2 Practice problems

I think we can certainly take advantage of some organizational synergy and increase our CAPEX rate if we approve this project.

1. Which of the following is the likely medium for the sentence above?

   A. Business memo

   B. Scientific journal

   C. Novel

   D. Motivational speech

2. Which of the following sentences would indicate that the setting is the United States in the 1920s?

   A. Rationing made our lives difficult, but we, like most citizens, were dedicated to the war effort.

   B. The local speakeasy was where he'd get his hooch when he had a few extra clams to spend.

   C. You could hear the clang of his riding spurs before the stranger pushed through the door of the saloon.

   D. She was a hep cat who had all the latest vinyl from the coolest bands around.

3. Perform an Internet search for examples of each of the following and make a list of three to five major conventions for each.

   A. Business letter

   B. Research paper

   C. Essay

E.2.3 *Apply basic knowledge of the elements of the writing process.*

Writing is not easy. Even the best writers can suffer from agonizing cases of writer's block, and making oneself clear often requires arduous rounds of revisions. Thankfully, there are plenty of tools and resources available to writers to assist in the process. This TEAS task will require you to be familiar with the writing process and the tools that writers employ in that process. What steps do they take? How do they organize the information? There are a multitude of great sources, many of them free on the Internet.

There might be nearly as many writing processes as there are writers, but in its basic form the process is made up of three steps: prewriting, writing, and revision. These steps are not necessarily distinct, and each writer will approach them in his or her own way. However, there are elements of each about which you should be knowledgeable.

Prewriting includes all the tasks necessary to start putting pen to paper (or, more likely, fingers to keyboard) and do the actual writing. This can include tasks as basic as determining when and where to write. Most professional writers set schedules to ensure that they are, at the very least, thinking about the piece they want to write. For any given piece, one of the first steps is to determine the thesis. That includes not just the topic, but also the purpose for writing about the topic. Brainstorming techniques, such as stream of consciousness writing or mind mapping, can be useful in finding a topic or a purpose.

Once the topic and purpose have been identified, the writer determines what research is needed. Depending on the type of writing, this could include nothing more than some time alone to think (personal essay), or it could require an assortment of primary and secondary sources that the author will need to cite within the finished piece. The research process will provide the material with which the writer will work. The next challenge is to organize that material into a coherent, engaging framework. Many writers use an outline to assist in organizing thoughts and constructing their pieces. Outlines create a hierarchy of information that allows writers to show coordination and subordination among related topics. In the example below, the writer is creating coordination between the main points of choosing ingredients and understanding cooking techniques. He's also indicating subordinate examples to cover for each main point.

> ## Taking Your Cooking to the Next Level
>
> I. Choosing your ingredients
>
>   a. Spices
>
>   b. Vegetables
>
>   c. Meats
>
> II. Understanding cooking techniques
>
>   a. Searing
>
>   b. Poaching
>
>   c. Slow roasting

This objective includes, but is not limited to, the following examples of knowledge, skills, and abilities.

- *Know elements of the writing process (e.g., planning/ preparation/outline, drafting, referencing sources, revision).*
- *Identify steps necessary to complete a writing task.*
- *Identify when citation is needed.*

Key terms

brainstorming. Discussing as a group to create an idea or solve a problem.

citation. A strictly formatted line of text that provides a source reference.

draft. An unfinished version of a text.

mind mapping. Visually diagramming ideas around a central concept.

stream of consciousness writing. A narrative device that mimics interior monologue.

ENGLISH

While the tasks previously mentioned could be considered prewriting, they often go on throughout the writing process. Most writers continue to discover new insights into their topics and purposes as they write, which creates a cycle of research and organization. Furthermore, the writing and revision processes are often indistinguishable. While some writers will complete a full first draft before revising, many writers revise as they write, constantly tinkering with their sentences. The process for people other than the writer to edit or proofread is likewise dependent upon the writer, the type of writing, and the publisher. For a professionally published piece of writing, there typically will be reviews by copy editors, fact checkers, and/or proofreaders with the chance for the writer to revise based on feedback. In some cases, the editors working for the publisher might have the final say on whether to revise something.

E.2.3 Practice problems

1. Which of the following situations requires the inclusion of a citation?

   A. The author made up the information.

   B. The author wants to emphasize the information.

   C. The author is giving an opinion.

   D. The author is quoting a source.

2. If all the following tasks are used in writing, which of the following would likely occur first?

   A. Interviewing potential sources

   B. Brainstorming interesting topics and organization

   C. Developing an organizational outline

   D. Ensuring proper citations

3. Find a magazine article that interests you and organize the article content into an outline. What are the coordinating main points? What are the subordinate topics below each main point?

E.2.4 *Develop a well-organized paragraph.*

Just as a sentence is the foundational unit of a complete thought, a paragraph is a self-contained unit of discourse and the building block for longer works of writing. A paragraph should convey a coherent message through all included sentences. To succeed on this TEAS task, you need to understand the conventions of good paragraph development, including the use of topic sentences, supporting details, and conclusions. You should be able to identify paragraph development strategies and areas where revision is required. Focusing on the coherence of the message will be the key to your success for this task.

While a paragraph can be as short as a single sentence, we'll focus mostly on longer examples that include the various parts of a well-constructed paragraph. First up is the topic sentence, which introduces, in a general way, the message or idea of the paragraph. A well-constructed paragraph requires adequate development in the form of supporting details that provide more specific information about the topic. A conclusion is used to sum up the idea, and often transitions are used to prepare for the introduction of a new idea. Take the following example.

Topic sentence	I'll never forget my English teacher, Ms. Miller, and her obsession with the notion of perfectly constructed paragraphs.
Supporting details	She insisted that every paragraph have at least five sentences, including a deftly wrought topic sentence with eloquent supporting details and a tidy conclusion.
	For a mere passing grade, we had to slave over every sentence to ensure that it contributed precisely to the unity of the message.
Conclusion/ transition	Needless to say, she wasn't the most popular teacher at the school, but we knew that we had her to thank for our eventual adventures in literature.

Search online for "types of paragraphs," and you'll quickly find that there's no consensus on the precise categories of paragraph construction. The main point is that the information is presented in a logical way. The example above, for instance, demonstrates a cause-and-effect paragraph construction. For cause and effect, the paragraph starts with a proposition (the teacher obsessed with paragraph writing) and lead the reader through the supporting details (the teacher's requirements, the students' efforts) to the effect (the students' improved writing). Another construct that might show up on the TEAS is chronological order, in which the time sequence guides the message. An emphasis paragraph is typically a short paragraph used to draw attention to an important or interesting message within the flow of the larger piece. A short emphasis paragraph can also be used as a transition. Evaluating various ways that paragraphs can present information cogently is a good exercise to prepare for this TEAS task.

This objective includes, but is not limited to, the following examples of knowledge, skills, and abilities.

- *Know the parts of a paragraph (e.g., topic sentence, supporting details, transitions, conclusion).*
- *Be able to put information in a logical order (e.g., chronological, emphasis, cause/effect).*
- *Identify information that does not belong.*
- *Identify where more information/development is needed.*

Key terms

emphasis paragraph. A short paragraph that highlights a key point.

supporting detail. Information that supports the main idea by answering who, what, where, when, or why.

topic sentence. The sentence that summarizes the main idea of a piece of text.

transition. Words or sentences that lead from one idea to another.

ENGLISH

When you're well-practiced at evaluating paragraph construction, it won't be difficult to notice some of the common problems that writers run into when writing paragraphs. One common trouble spot is the inclusion of information that doesn't support the topic of the paragraph. If the sentence makes you stop and reread, maybe it should not have been included in this particular paragraph. Ask yourself, "How does this contribute to the topic and the rest of the paragraph?" Another problem is when vital information has been omitted. This also might make you stop to reread. Would a transition have helped? What information would clarify the message of the paragraph? It's often helpful to determine what principle is being used to organize the information and then determine what's required for that principle to work best.

E.2.4 Practice problems

1. Which of the following examples would most likely act as a transition sentence?

   A. I find that older modes of technology often appeal to me in ways I can't quite articulate.

   B. The tap-tap-tap of a typewriter, for instance, inspires my creative writing impulses.

   C. The rich, warm sound of a vinyl record makes me want to throw out all my CDs.

   D. I suppose it could be nostalgia, but I suspect that it might be something else.

   I. By the time I made it to the bus stop, I was starting to feel a bit of a cold coming on.

   II. After a quick, regrettably cold shower, I shoveled a bowl of cereal in my mouth while simultaneously getting caught up on email.

   III. Twenty minutes later, when I walked into the office, I was undeniably sick.

   IV. My day started, unfortunately, with a 6 a.m. alarm that would resound in my head until I mercifully fell asleep 12 hours later.

2. Which of the following is the best chronological sequence to construct a paragraph with these sentences?

   A. IV, II, I, III

   B. IV, III, II, I

   C. I, II, III, IV

   D. I, III, IV, II

3. Write three paragraphs using the following table to organize the sentences.

Topic sentence		
Supporting details		
Conclusion/transition		

Practice problem answers

E.2.1

1. Option B is correct. The first verb is in the past tense, while the verb for the second independent clause is in the present tense. Using "and" is an appropriate choice to demonstrate agreement between the ideas of an intrepid traveler being unable to keep her from taking a trip. Poor diction and ambiguous word choice are incorrect because the words selected for use in this sentence fit the context and convey a clear message.

2. Option C is correct. This is a good choice to indicate that the second idea is an effect of the first idea.
   - Using "although" indicates opposition between the two ideas, while the context points toward effect.
   - Using "in other words" indicates an example, while the context points toward effect.
   - Using "meanwhile" provides a time relationship between the two ideas, which is not the best transition to use for this context.

E.2.2

1. Option A is correct. This passage contains jargon (synergy, CAPEX rate) that would be commonly understood within a business setting.
   - The jargon in this passage would not likely be found in a scientific journal.
   - The jargon in the passage would not likely be found in a novel, unless that novel focused on a business environment.
   - The passage doesn't contain any motivational techniques.

2. Option B is correct. The slang and the reference to a Prohibition-era speakeasy indicate that the setting for this passage is the 1920s.
   - The references in option A point to World War II, which the United States participated in during the 1940s.
   - The reference to riding spurs and a saloon indicates that the setting for this was during the "Old West."
   - The slang from option D would be more appropriate for the 1940s or later.

E.2.3

1. Option D is correct. Quoting a source, whether published or unpublished, requires inclusion of a citation.
   - Fictional events do not require citations.
   - The need for citation is not related to emphasis.
   - Opinions do not require citation.

2. Option B is correct. This would likely be the first step that would guide the research and organization.
   - This research wouldn't be conducted until the topic had been determined.
   - The organization likely wouldn't occur until the topic had been determined.
   - Ensuring proper citations wouldn't occur until after the research had been conducted.

E.2.4

1. Option D is correct. The second part of this sentence is vague, which is a good means for transitioning to another paragraph that will flesh out what "something else" refers to.
   - Option A is the topic sentence, and it introduces rather than transitions.
   - Options B and C are supporting details and don't provide a transition.

2. Option A is correct. This sequence makes the most sense, starting with the alarm, followed by breakfast, the bus stop, and work.

E.3.1 *Use context clues to determine the meaning of words or phrases.*

Perhaps you've heard the phrase "context is everything"? Well, for this particular TEAS task, that is certainly the case. You will use context clues to determine the correct meaning of words and phrases. That context can come from tone, other words or ideas within the sentence, or the larger overall context of a passage. You'll be asked to evaluate context and choose the meaning that best matches it from a list of options.

One fairly straightforward way to determine the meaning of a word or phrase is to evaluate the surrounding text for clues. For example, if a word is presented in a series, its meaning should fit with the meaning of the other words in a series. You wouldn't confuse the word "shake" in the series "burgers, fries, and a shake" with a handshake. Synonyms can also provide clues about intended meaning. Take the word "break," which has a number of different meanings. The sentence below demonstrates how a synonym can clue you in.

> I always felt that he just needed an opportunity, and this project proved to be the break he needed.

The preceding mention of "opportunity" should provide the context that this instance of "break" refers to a chance to achieve success.

Sometimes, though, you'll have to pick up on more subtle clues dealing with tone or logical inferences about constructions such as cause and effect. See if you can find the cause and effect in another example using the word "break."

> She had suffered through a run of difficult, time-consuming projects, and this project proved to be the break she needed.

In this case, there is no synonym or series to guide you. Based on the context, though, of numerous "difficult and time-consuming projects" (cause), we can infer that this instance of "break" refers to a needed respite (effect). In some cases, the setting can provide the clue needed to determine the correct word. If we know, for instance, that the setting is a ship at sea, then we can easily determine that a reference to a "log" probably does not mean a portion of a fallen tree but rather a record of a trip.

While a good vocabulary will prove helpful to succeed at this task, it's not necessary to start reading the dictionary. What's more important is practicing careful reading and being able to find the clues within context. You might not even need to know the definitions of a given word to answer these questions correctly. If the question provides options, try each of those out within the context. Which one seems to work the best? Attempt to figure out what makes the most sense based on what is known from the passage.

This objective includes, but is not limited to, the following examples of knowledge, skills, and abilities.

- *Know synonyms.*
- *Be aware of tone.*
- *Associate words in a series.*
- *Recognize cause and effect.*
- *Be aware of general ideas of a passage.*

Key terms

context. Surrounding words that lend meaning to an idea.

synonyms. Words with identical or similar meanings.

tone. The implied attitude toward the topic.

E.3.1 Practice problems

After a couple of failures, he turned his efforts in a new direction.

1. Which of the following is the meaning of the word "turn" in the example?
   - A. To reverse the position of
   - B. To get beyond
   - C. To deflect
   - D. To apply

2. In which of the following sentences does "runs" mean "manages"?
   - A. The car runs on diesel.
   - B. The road runs the length of the island.
   - C. She runs the department efficiently.
   - D. His son runs the streets like a grown up.

3. Perform an Internet search for "words with multiple meanings." Pick five words. Write two or three sentences for each word, using different contexts to employ different meanings for that word.

E.3.2 *Determine the meaning of words by analyzing word parts.*

This objective includes, but is not limited to, the following examples of knowledge, skills, and abilities.

- *Know common affixes.*
  - *Prefixes: anti-, dys-, inter-, intra-, mid-, pre-, non- sub-, super-, un-*
  - *Suffixes: -ful, ic, -ation, -ology, -ness, -ous*
- *Combine affixes with root words.*

Key terms

affix. Letters placed at the beginning or end of a word or word part to change its meaning.

derivation. Determining the origin of a word.

inflection. Details of how a word is expressed to modify its tone or meaning.

morpheme. The smallest meaningful unit in grammar.

prefix. An affix that appears at the beginning of a word.

root. A word to which an affix can be attached.

suffix. An affix that appears at the end of a word.

The English language can be a lot like social networking: Knowing one word (or person) easily leads you to countless others. That is especially the case when you familiarize yourself with morphemes, or word parts. Morphemes are the smallest grammatical unit of meaning, and affixes are morphemes that are attached to a word stem, or root, to form either a new word or a grammatical variation of the same word. For this TEAS task, you need to be able to expand your network by taking the word parts you know and evaluating how they can alter meaning or contribute to new meanings. You should review lists of common prefixes and suffixes and study how they are paired with various root words and complex bases.

Let's start at the beginning—of the word, that is—with prefixes. Prefixes are added to the beginning of a stem to create new meaning. There are innumerable lists of prefixes available to review on the Internet, and it's a good idea to browse some of these lists. Here is a short one just to whet your appetite.

Prefix	Meaning	Example	Example meaning
a-	not	asymmetric	not symmetric
epi-	on, above	epidural	outside the dura mater
hyper-	a lot; too much	hypercalcemia	too much calcium in the blood
hypo-	a little; not enough	hypokalemia	not enough potassium in the blood
supra-	above	supraorbital	above the eye sockets

There are some principles you should keep in mind as well. Some prefixes, for example, can only be added to particular parts of speech. For instance, re-, meaning "again," should only be added to verb bases. When evaluating word parts, be sure to reflect on whether the meaning of an affix makes sense to use with the base. Another consideration for prefixes is whether to use a hyphen. In most cases, the prefix should be added without using a hyphen, but there are exceptions. Guidelines you should know include the following.

Guideline	Example
Hyphenate prefixes before proper nouns or proper adjectives.	trans-Siberian mid-America
Hyphenate all words beginning with self-, ex-, and all-.	self-made ex-president all-around
Hyphenate when it adds clarity.	re-cover (cover again) vs. recover (recuperate)

Hyphenation is not an issue for suffixes, which—you guessed it—are placed after the stem. They might not change the word's meaning. In fact, many of the most commonly used and understood suffixes do not form new words, but rather express different grammatical categories (tense, number, etc.). Here's a brief list of inflectional suffixes and what they express.

Suffix	Action
-s, -es, -ies	plural
-ed	past tense
-ing	progressive/continuous
-er	comparative
-est	superlative

You'll also want to be familiar with derivational suffixes, or those that form new words when added to the stem. These can be divided into two categories: those that change the part of speech (class-changing) and those that don't (class-maintaining).

Suffix	Action
-ise, -ize	usually changes nouns into verbs
-ly	usually changes adjectives into adverbs
-able, -ible	usually changes verbs into adjectives
-ist	class-maintaining, retained in a noun
-logy, -ology	class-maintaining, retained in a noun

Becoming familiar with a range of affixes and roots—particularly those used commonly in medical settings—should help you succeed on this TEAS task. You might not know the exact meaning of a given word, but if you notice that the prefix anti- is attached, you'll at least have a clue that this word means "against" something. That might be all the information you need to direct you toward the right answer.

E.3.2 Practice problems

1. In which of the following words does the suffix create a word different from the root version?

   A. Handful

   B. Defended

   C. Hiding

   D. Runs

2. Based on an examination of the word parts, which of the following means "slow heart rate"?

   A. Bradycardia

   B. Bradypnea

   C. Tachycardia

   D. Tachypnea

3. Perform an Internet search for "medical roots, prefixes, and suffixes" and choose a site with a good list. Review the list and make mental note of the roots and affixes you know. Type up a list of those you have seen regularly but couldn't define.

Practice problem answers

E.3.1

1. Option D is correct. This is the best definition for this context, which is evident by replacing the word "turned" with "applied" in the sentence.

2. Option C is correct. The context of "the department" indicates that this use of "runs" means "to manage."
   - In option A, "runs" means "to operate."
   - In option B, "runs" means "to extend."
   - In option D, "runs" means "to go about freely."

E.3.2

1. Option A is correct. The suffix -ful changes the root "hand" to another word indicating an amount.
   - The suffix -ed changes the tense but does not create a new word.
   - The suffix -ing changes the tense but does not create a new word.
   - The suffix -s changes the number but does not create a new word.

2. Option A is correct. The prefix brady- means slow, and the stem cardia refers to the heart.
   - The stem pnea refers to breathing.
   - The prefix tachy- means fast.
   - The prefix tachy- means fast, and the stem pnea refers to breathing.

English section quiz

It occurred to me, a little too late, that leaving knifes on the counter with intrepid children around was a dangerous oversight.

1. Which of the following is misspelled in the sentence?
   A. occurred
   B. knifes
   C. intrepid
   D. oversight

It's probably too late, but I would still like to try to make it to the museum, including the special exhibition; try the food at that bar and grill, and take a walk along the pier.

2. Which of the following punctuation marks is used incorrectly in the sentence?
   A. The apostrophe in the word "It's"
   B. The comma after the word "late"
   C. The semicolon after the word "exhibition"
   D. The comma after the word "grill"

Cooking delicious meals literally requires you to be worth your salt.

3. Which of the following is the complete predicate in the sentence?
   A. Cooking
   B. Cooking delicious meals
   C. requires
   D. literally requires

4. Which of the following is a simple sentence?
   A. The woman who looked out of place.
   B. Looked out of place in the evening store.
   C. The woman in the convenience store looked out of place since she was dressed for an evening out.
   D. The woman in the elegant, gold evening gown and diamond-studded tiara looked out of place in the convenience store.

5. Which of the following nouns is written in the correct plural form?
   A. data
   B. crisises
   C. formula
   D. mooses

6. Which of the following sentences would most likely be found in an academic research paper on psychiatry?
   A. He stalked ominously back and forth across his doctor's office, muttering incoherently.
   B. The researcher felt that he had struck the mother lode when he came across his subject's personal papers.
   C. He collected the data with an admirable amount of fieldwork.
   D. The subjects participated in a double-blind study focused on long-term outcomes.

7. Which of the following sentences makes the best topic sentence?
   A. Not only did the two teams combine for several outstanding goals, but the physicality of the play was exceptional.
   B. Needless to say, no one left the stadium without some memories to share.
   C. The match was filled with enough drama to keep the fans talking about it for days.
   D. Not a single player conceded an inch of the field.

Wow, I can't believe he's strutting with so much swag after being rejected so harshly.

8. Which of the following words from the sentence is slang?
   A. Wow
   B. can't
   C. swag
   D. harshly

9. Which of the following sentences has correct subject-verb agreement?
   A. When the cafeteria serves lime gelatin for lunch, each of the children asks for more.
   B. As the car lurches forward, every one of the passengers brace for the impact.
   C. Because the bus broke down on the way, the group of swimmers are late to the meet.
   D. In this scenario, the family of four miss the flight because there was not enough parking at the airport.

The young girl felt the sting of unfairness at being—as she felt—framed by her little brother.

10. Which of the following is the best synonym for "framed" as used in the sentence?
    A. Incriminated
    B. Conceived
    C. Constructed
    D. Uttered

ENGLISH

> Apparently I needed my morning coffee because I was being obtuse despite my best efforts to grasp the concepts we covered in class that morning.

11. Which of the following is an appropriate synonym for "obtuse" as used in the sentence?
    A. Blunt
    B. Uncomprehending
    C. Insensitive
    D. Crass

> The ignoble manner in which our stepmother treated us was unfair and made us feel like we were nothing to her.

12. Which of the following best captures the meaning of "ignoble" as used in the sentence?
    A. Sarcastic
    B. Impatient
    C. Demeaning
    D. Manipulative

13. Which of the following words is an exception to a common spelling rule?
    A. Batted
    B. Lives
    C. Albeit
    D. Believe

> Our parents gave us an ultimatum_ Do exactly as they instructed or spend the rest of the summer grounded.

14. Which of the following punctuation marks best completes the sentence?
    A. .
    B. ,
    C. ;
    D. :

> The goat was incredibly agile as it scampered along the ridge.

15. Which of the following parts of speech is "incredibly" as used in the sentence?
    A. Verb
    B. Adverb
    C. Adjective
    D. Interjection

16. Which of the following is correctly punctuated?
    A. Due to the time-sensitive nature of the request the lawyer faxed the document to the judge.
    B. Due to the time-sensitive nature of the request. The lawyer had faxed the document to the judge.
    C. Due to the time-sensitive nature of the request, the lawyer faxed the document to the judge.
    D. Due to the time-sensitive nature of the request; the lawyer had faxed the document to the judge.

17. Which of the following examples is a complete sentence?
    A. Believe it.
    B. On the topic of love.
    C. Whether you want it or not.
    D. Despite my best efforts and persistence.

I. Basketball Strategy
   A. Offense
      1. Isolation plays
      2. Motion offense
      3. Special situations
   B. Defense
      1. Man-to-man
      2. Zone
      3. Special situations

18. Which of the following statements is true regarding this outline?
    A. Motion offense is a type of isolation play.
    B. Man-to-man defense takes precedence over zone defense.
    C. Basketball strategy can be subdivided into offense and defense.
    D. Special situations use the same strategies for both offense and defense.

19. Which of the following sentences is irrelevant as part of a paragraph composed of these sentences?
    A. Our ultimate goal was to win a championship, and we practiced tirelessly to that end.
    B. Most days, we were up before dawn to work on conditioning before starting drills.
    C. Our coach devised an ingenious strategy that we knew would give us a competitive advantage.
    D. We knew that hard work and sweat would be the keys to our success.

20. Which of the following phrases follows the rules of capitalization?
    A. Professor Hopping
    B. Thanksgiving day
    C. uncle Larry
    D. Northern Canada

> I lost my book bag.
>
> My book bag contained my lunch money.
>
> I was very hungry.
>
> I had a difficult time staying awake in class that afternoon.

21. Which of the following options best uses grammar to combine the sentences for clarity and readability?
    A. I was very hungry because I lost my book bag. It contained my lunch money, and it was difficult to stay awake in class that afternoon.
    B. Because I lost my book bag that contained my lunch money, I was very hungry in the afternoon and had a difficult time staying awake in class.
    C. It was difficult to stay awake in class that afternoon, because I lost my lunch money. It was in my book bag, and I was very hungry.
    D. My book bag contained my lunch money, and I lost it. I was so hungry that afternoon that I had a difficult time staying awake in class.

22. Which of the following prefixes should be added to a word function to indicate something that is not functioning well?
   A. anti–
   B. dys–
   C. non–
   D. sub–

23. Based on an analysis of the word parts, which of the following means "water on the brain"?
   A. Hypercephalus
   B. Hydrocephalus
   C. Hypomania
   D. Hypnomania

   The client made an appointment with a cosmetic surgeon to discuss possible rhinoplasty.

24. In the sentence, the prefix rhino– in the word "rhinoplasty" indicates that this client is interested in cosmetic surgery related to which of the following?
   A. Eyes
   B. Chin
   C. Forehead
   D. Nose

English section quiz rationales

1. Option B is correct. The plural of "knife" follows the rule of changing -f or -fe to -ves. Thus, the word should be spelled "knives." Option A is the correct spelling for the past tense of the word "occur." It follows the rule to double the final consonant. Option C is the correct spelling for the word meaning fearless. Option D is the correct spelling for the word meaning an unintentional failure to consider. See E.1.1 for related information.

2. Option D is correct. Because one of the items in this list includes a comma, semicolons should be used to separate the items. Option A is an appropriate use of an apostrophe to form a conjunction. Option B is an appropriate use of a comma to separate two independent clauses. Option C is an appropriate use of a semicolon to separate items in a list if one of them contains commas. See E.1.2 for related information.

3. Option D is correct. This is the complete predicate, which includes the simple predicate and its modifiers. Option A is a gerund, or a verb acting as a noun. It is the simple subject of the sentence. Option B is the complete subject. Option C is the simple predicate. See E.1.3 for related information.

4. Option D is correct. It is constructed as a simple sentence containing one subject and one verb. Options A and B are not complete sentences. Option C contains a dependent clause, making it complex. See E.1.3 for related information.

5. Option A is correct. Data is the plural form of datum, meaning a piece of information. The plural form of crisis is crises. The plural forms of formula are formulas and formulae. The plural form of moose is moose. See E.1.2 for related information.

6. Option D is correct. The neutral tone and the context of "subjects" and "double-blind study" make this the most likely example to be found in an academic research paper on psychiatry. The descriptive language of Option A ("stalked," "ominously") is not typical of a research paper. The use of slang in Option B ("struck the mother lode") would likely be avoided in a research paper. The value word "admirable" in Option C is not typical of a research paper. See E.2.2 for related information.

7. Option C is correct. This sentence is the best example of the type of introductory information expected from a topic sentence. Option A would better serve as a supporting detail to a topic sentence. Option B would better serve as a summary sentence given the lack of context provided. Option D would better serve as a supporting detail to a topic sentence. See E.2.4 for related information.

8. Option C is correct. This usage of "swag" is slang meaning self-confidence or swagger. "Wow" is an interjection, usually an exclamation of surprise, which is not the same as slang. A contraction is not necessarily slang. The adverb "harshly" is used according to its standard meaning. See E.2.2 for related information.

9. Option A is correct. The subject "each" should take a singular verb, as it does here with "asks." The subject "one" in Option B should take a singular verb, but in this case the verb "brace" is plural. The subject "group" in Option C should take a singular verb, but in this case the verb "are" is plural. The subject "family" in Option D should take a singular verb, but in this case the verb "miss" is plural. See E.2.1 for related information.

10. Option A is correct. The idea of incrimination best fits the context of someone who felt unfairness. Options B, C, and D do not best fit the context of the sentence. See E.3.1 for related information.

11. Option B is correct. Given the context of an inability to grasp concepts, "uncomprehending" is the best synonym for "obtuse" in this sentence. While "blunt," "insensitive," and "crass" can be synonyms for "obtuse," they do not fit the context of being unable to grasp concepts. See E.3.1 for related information.

12. Option C is correct. Within this context, the word "ignoble" is used to describe a manner of treatment that is demeaning and employed to make one feel less worthy. This is strengthened by the contextual clue "made us feel like we were nothing to her." Although "sarcastic," "impatient," and "manipulative" fit the tone of the sentence, they do not mean the same thing as "ignoble." See E.3.1 for related information.

13. Option C is correct. This spelling is an exception to the I before E rule. Option A is the correct spelling for the past tense of the word "bat." It follows the rule to double the final consonant. The plural of "life" in Option B follows the rule of changing -f or -fe to -ves. Option D follows the I before E rule. See E.1.1 for related information.

14. Option D is correct. A colon can be used to introduce a clause that illustrates a preceding clause, as in this sentence. A period would create two separate sentences, which is not the best way to indicate that the second clause illustrates the first clause. A comma should not be used separate two independent clauses. While a semicolon can be used to separate independent clauses, it is not the best means for conveying the relationship between these clauses. See E.1.2 for related information.

15. Option B is correct. The word "incredibly" modifies the adjective "agile" and is thus an adverb. A verb is an action word, which is not how "incredibly" is used here. An adjective modifies a noun, and that is not how "incredibly" is used here. An interjection is a word used to a particular emotion, which is not how "incredibly" is used here. See E.1.3 for related information.

16. Option C is correct. An introductory clause like the one used in this sentence should be set off with a comma. See E.1.2 for related information.

17. Option A is correct. The understood "you" is the subject, and "believe" is the predicate. They combine to create a complete thought. Options B, C, and D do not include a subject and a predicate. See E.2.1 for related information.

18. Option C is correct. Offense and defense are at the same level under basketball strategy, so it follows that these are subdivisions of the main topic. Motion offense and isolation plays are two different types of offense. Just because man-to-man defense is listed first doesn't necessarily indicate a value judgment or precedence. While special situations are listed for both offense and defense, they do not necessarily use the same strategies. See E.2.3 for related information.

19. Option C is correct. This sentence does not fit the topic of practicing tirelessly toward the championship goal. Option A is an acceptable topic sentence for this paragraph. Option B is an appropriate supporting detail for the topic sentence. Option D is an appropriate summary for the topic sentence. See E.2.4 for related information.

20. Option A is correct. A person's title is capitalized when it appears before his or her name. In Option B, the full title of a holiday should be capitalized. In Option C, "uncle" is used as a title and should be capitalized. In Option D, "northern" is used as an adjective rather than as part of the place name and should not be capitalized. See E.2.1 for related information.

21. Option B is correct. This option is an example of the use of grammar to enhance clarity and readability. The four sentences are combined into one clear, succinct sentence that is easy to read and understand. While the grammar is correct, Options A, C, and D do not clearly express the writer's intent. See E.2.1 for related information.

22. Option B is correct. This prefix means "ill" or "bad," which is the best choice to indicate poor function. Option A means "against," which is not the best way to indicate that something is not functioning properly. Option C means "not," which would indicate no functionality. Option D means "below," which could indicate decreased functionality but is not the best choice. See E.3.2 for related information.

23. Option B is correct. The prefix "hydro" refers to water, and the stem "cephalus" refers to the head or brain. Option A is not an actual word, but based on the word parts would mean "excessive head." The prefix "hypo" in Option C means "below," and the stem "mania" refers to an obsessive preoccupation. The prefix "hypno" in Option D refers to sleep, and the stem "mania" refers to an obsessive preoccupation. See E.3.2 for related information.

24. Option D is correct. The prefix rhino- refers to the nose. The stem plasty refers to surgical repair. The prefix oculo- refers to the eyes. The prefix mento- refers to the chin. The prefix front- refers to the forehead. See E.3.2 for related information.